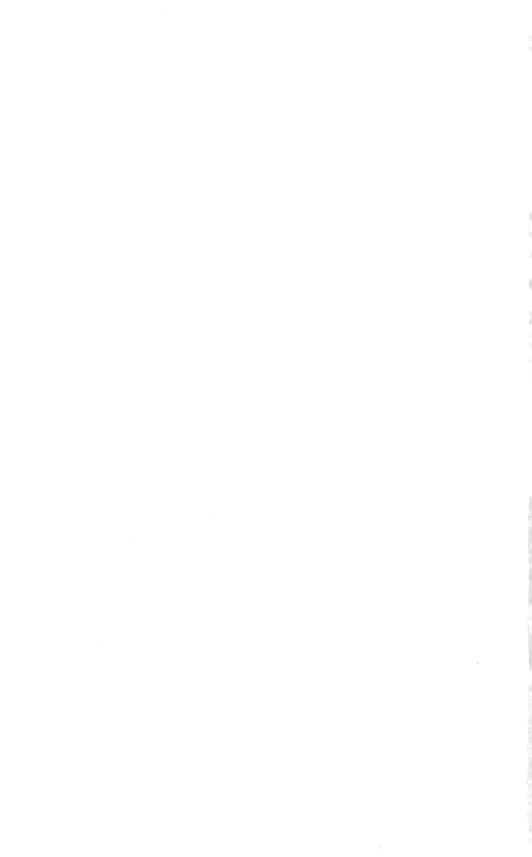

Springer Series on Advanced Practice Nursing

Terry T. Fulmer, PhD, C, FAAN, Series Editor
New York University School of Nursing

Advisory Board: Joyce Anastasi, RN, PhD; Susan Kelly, RN, PhD, FAAN; Tish Knobf, MSN, RN, FAAN; Mairead Hickey, RN, PhD

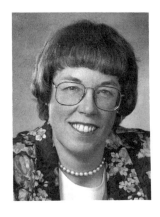

Barbara J. Daly, PhD, RN, FAAN, received her bachelor of science in nursing from the University of Massachusetts, her master's in nursing from Case Western Reserve University, and her doctorate in philosophy from Bowling Green State University. Dr. Daly's primary faculty appointment is in the School of Nursing at Case Western Reserve University, where she also holds secondary appointments in the School of Medicine and the Center for Biomedical Ethics. Her clinical background is in critical care nursing and she is currently the Director of the Acute Care Nurse Practitioner program at the Frances Payne Bolton School of Nursing, CWRU. In addition, she serves as Co-Director of the Clinical Ethics Service at University Hospitals of Cleveland. She has spoken at national and international conferences and published widely in the areas of clinical ethics, innovative nursing practice models, and the development of the Acute Care Nurse Practitioner role.

THE ACUTE CARE NURSE PRACTITIONER

Barbara J. Daly, PhD, RN, FAAN

Editor

Springer Publishing Company

Springer Publishing Company, Inc.
536 Broadway
New York, NY 10012-3955

Cover design by Margaret Dunin
Production Editor: Kathleen Kelly

97 98 99 00 01 / 6 5 4 3 2

Library of Congress Cataloging-in-Publication Data
The acute care nurse practitioner / Barbara J. Daly, editor.
     p. cm.—(Springer series on advanced practice nursing)
    Includes bibliographical references and index.
    ISBN 0-8261-9480-X
    1. Intensive care nursing. 2. Nurse practitioners. I. Daly,
Barbara J. II. Series: The Springer series on advanced practice
nursing.
    [DNLM: 1. Nurse Practitioners. 2. Acute Disease—nursing.
WY 129 A189 1997]
RT120.I5A338   1997
510.73′61—DC21
DNLM/DLC
for Library of Congress   96-46566
                                        CIP

Printed in the United States of America

CONTENTS

CONTRIBUTORS

John M. Clochesy, PhD, RN, CS, FAAN, FCCM, is an Associate Professor of Nursing in the Department of Acute and Tertiary Care and is also an Assistant Dean of the School of Nursing at the University of Pittsburgh.

Anne M. Gedwill, MSN, ND, RN, CS, is an Acute Care Nurse Practitioner in an adult Hematology/Oncology division at University Hospitals of Cleveland.

Carol A. Genet, MS, RN, CS, is an Instructor of Nursing in the Acute Care Nurse Practitioner Program at the Frances Payne Bolton School of Nursing at Case Western Reserve University. She is also an Adult Nurse Practitioner.

Sharon Mack, MSN, RN, CS, is an Acute Care Nurse Practitioner on a medical division at University Hospitals of Cleveland, where she provides direct patient care within a collaborative practice model.

Diane K. Mlakar, MSN, RN, is an Acute Care Nurse Practitioner on an adult Neurology division and Intensive Care Unit managing stroke patients at University Hospitals of Cleveland.

Kathleen Parrinello, PhD, RN, is Senior Director for Hospital Operations and directs all hospital clinical and support programs at the University of Rochester, Strong Memorial Hospital and is an Associate Professor of Clinical Nursing at the University of Rochester School of Nursing and also teaches nursing administration.

Jean E. Steel, PhD, FAAN, is an Associate Professor, School of Nursing at the University of Connecticut and coordinates the Primary Care Nurse Practitioner Program.

Helen Stupak Shah, DNSc, RN, is an Associate Professor at the University of Connecticut School of Nursing where she coordinates the Acute Care Nurse Practitioner Program.

Rachel K. Vanek, RNC, MSN, is an Acute Care Nurse Practitioner in the Medical Intensive Care Unit at University Hospitals at Cleveland.

Chapter **1**

INTRODUCTION: A VISION FOR THE ACUTE CARE NURSE PRACTITIONER ROLE

Barbara J. Daly, PhD, RN, FAAN

This work is intended to be both a report and a guideline. It is a report of the conditions and events associated with the recent initiation and development of a direct care role for advanced practice nurses in acute care settings—the acute care nurse practitioner (ACNP) role. It is a guideline for educators involved in starting ACNP programs, for administrators considering hiring ACNPs, and for ACNPs themselves as they prepare for practice. The need to provide a single document that serves both functions at once reflects the rapidity with which this role has developed.

The format of the book follows stages in the development of this role. The history of the nurse practitioner (NP) movement will be briefly reviewed by Steel in chapter 2 to provide the background from which this new role for practitioners grew. Following this, a discussion of trends in acute care will assist the reader in understanding the forces that have created both the opportunity and need for ACNPs. With any new role, much of the work of the profession must

1

focus on designing and implementing appropriate educational programs, and chapters 4 and 5 discuss both the program or didactic
components and the clinical preparation. Once educated, of course,
ACNPs must find a role for themselves in an acute care facility.
Parrinello lends insight to the perspective of the nurse administrator
and describes the practice model for ACNPs at a tertiary-care facility. Last, ACNPs from one of the first educational programs
describe their experience in actually implementing the role.

Prior to offering these specific discussions, it may be helpful to
clarify the philosophy and assumptions of the authors. Although
there is little doubt that the ACNP role plays a major part in
nursing education today and that this role is gaining increased
acceptance by hospital administrators, there will be significant
variation in how the purpose and functions of the role are understood. Therefore, this introduction will briefly present our beliefs
about the genesis of the role and the mission of acute care nurse
practitioners.

ORIGINS OF THE ROLE

It is important to understand that ACNP educational programs
arose not from any particular planning efforts or consensus within
the profession, but simply as a response to a demand. The current
environment of acute care created a need that, in the current climate
of rather desperate attempts to keep health care systems going, led
to a demand for a new practitioner. This demand was followed by the
professional response and hurried agreement about the appropriateness of creating an advanced practice role that would address these
needs (Figure 1.1).

Much of the impetus for change in the current acute care system,
described in more detail in chapter 3, arises from a mismatch between characteristics of present practice models of both physicians
and nurses and patient needs. In addition, residency programs are
downsizing acute care residency positions as part of the national
focus on emphasizing primary care and generalist preparation. In
fact, the projected decrease in direct care providers, more than any

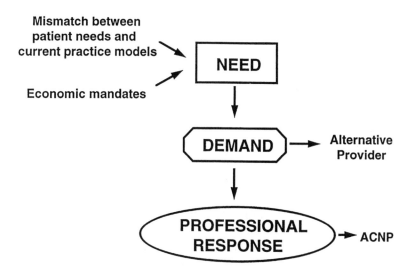

FIGURE 1.1 Genesis of the acute care practitioner.

commitment to alter the way in which care is delivered, has fueled the demand for an alternative provider.

This leads to the question, what kind of provider? The historical context regarding the ability of nurses to function in expanded roles provides the answer. We have a 30-year history now with the NP role, one that repeatedly has been demonstrated to be associated with reliable and high-quality care to patients as well as with reduced costs. We have almost as much history with use of advanced practice nurses (APNs) in the hospital. Clinical nurse specialists (CNSs), nurse midwives, and nurse anesthetists had become familiar sights by the 1980s. Additionally, some sporadic reports of trials of NPs in the inpatient setting were starting to appear in the literature as some facilities started to test this idea (Dale, 1991; Goksel, Harrison, Morrison, & Miller, 1993; Weinberg, Liljestrand, &Moore, 1983).

As so often happens, though, the real impetus for change came from the economic sector. It was not that the profession recognized and overtly agreed that NPs should have a role in the acute care hospital. It was more subtle than this, and perhaps more a recognition that *something* had to be done, that the current system was dysfunctional and inadequate. And into this gap came the ACNP.

RESPONSE

The professional response to this gap and the need for a new practitioner has been quite rapid. In the past few years there have been four clear stages of development that speak to the acuity of need and the ability of our profession to mobilize and respond.

First there were reports in the literature of some trial programs, describing local responses. The University of Pennsylvania, University of Connecticut, and Case Western Reserve University, for example, all published reports on their acute care or tertiary-care nurse practitioner programs (Clochesy, Daly, Idemoto, Steel, & Fitzpatrick, 1994; Keane & Richmond, 1993; Shah, Sullivan, Lattanzio, & Bruttomesso, 1993). Next, in short order, the need for a gathering of representatives from across the country who were interested in ACNP programs became evident and the first consensus conference was held. This conference was held in Boston in 1993 and was attended by 40 representatives from 21 facilities and organizations. A second conference was held in Cleveland in 1994, and this one was attended by 80 representatives from 31 facilities and organizations, from 21 states and from Canada. At that time there were 16 colleges and universities that had initiated acute care practitioner programs and another dozen or so in development. From these two meetings, a beginning consensus was established regarding the issues of titling, role, and curricular standards.

Next, using the consensus conference work as a basis, the American Nurses Association also responded rapidly. A Task Force was established in collaboration with the American Association of Critical Care Nurses (AACN), and a Scope of Practice document (American Association of Critical Care Nurses & American Nurses Association, 1995) was developed. This was crucial, not just as a policy statement about the profession's conception of this new role, but also as a basis for a credentialing procedure. After some continued negotiation between AACN and the American Nurses Credentialing Center (ANCC), it was agreed that the two organizations would work together to develop one certification exam to be offered through ANCC, so that ACNPs could become certified in the appropriate specialty. This is necessary, of course, for practice privileges in some states.

VISIONS

If the only purpose of the ACNP role was to be a substitute for interns and residents and to improve the efficiency of acute care, the job of preparing acute care practitioners would be fairly easy. We would simply take experienced acute care nurses, train them in technological procedures and treatment algorithms, and show them how to use care paths to get patients out of the hospital in the shortest time with the least variance from established standards. This would not be too difficult; however, it also would not be enough.

The conceptualization of the role that is described in this book reflects a vision that has three components. The best recognized function of the ACNP is assuredly to substitute for physicians, to deliver cost-effective bedside care. However, this function must be supplemented by fidelity to our duties as professional nurses and by a commitment to be part of a redesign of the fundamental way in which health care is and is not provided.

Improved Health Care / Professional Commitment

What saves us, as a discipline, from giving in to the temptation to take the easier road, to simply prepare physician extenders, is the realization that we always have an additional mission. We are not preparing just members of the work force; we are preparing professional nurses for advanced roles. These are critically different missions and it is this second mission that allows us to be quite comfortable in responding to skeptics who sincerely worry that we are giving up our professional ideals, that the ACNP is nothing more than a somewhat more efficient resident, and that we must sacrifice our essential nursing identity when we take over medical tasks.

Consideration of the characteristics and competencies of graduates of ACNP programs illustrates why this role is more than just a substitute. It is our professional identity and ideals that mandate that part of our mission must be to enable the graduate to provide care to patients that is more than diagnosis and intervention aimed at fixing organ pathology. In acute care and even in the most technologically sophisticated critical care units of tertiary-care centers, patients need nurses to help them define goals, choose alternatives, identify interventions that will address health problems in addition to physiologic dysfunction. Even in the midst of a physiologic crisis, patients need nurses to be thinking about and planning treatment regimens that will work at home, that will keep them out of these crises, that will fit into that patient's family structure, religion, culture, and capabilities. We are not trying to meet the need for someone just to write fluid orders and insert arterial lines; we want a practitioner who will restore patients to a state of health where they do not need acute care, a practitioner who can make the system more effective from the consumer point of view, and a practitioner who is skilled enough to surpass whatever barriers arise.

The profession of nursing will always have individual nurses who do not share this part of the vision. We have these people in all sorts of roles, and we will have ACNPs who do not see that they have a role beyond being members of the work force, meeting market demands. However, it is clear to us that this will not be the predominant view of our mission. Simply put, as nurses we have a moral commitment to do more than imitate medicine. As nurses, we will not stop affirming "the element of interpersonal connection between nurse and [patient] (American Nurses Association, 1995)." While it is clear that the emerging role of the ACNP is perfectly consistent with our nursing heritage and philosophy, it is crucial to be very clear when designing our programs and writing role descriptions that supporting advanced practitioners of the nursing profession, not just the health care work force, must be part of our mission.

PARTICIPATING IN HEALTH CARE REFORM

The third mission has implications for the curriculum of the ACNP tract as well as for overall graduate program design. We believe that we should go beyond the two visions described so far and have a clear commitment to a third—educating practitioners who will contribute to the continued evolution of the health care system. It is not enough to produce expert practitioners. We must have nurses prepared at the graduate level who are positioned to meet the needs of a reformed system. It would be a serious error to be so keen to meet the demand for case managers that we stop preparing CNSs, nurse managers, and educators, or that we inadvertently devalue these roles or make the mistake of thinking that one program can prepare nurses to perform all of these functions.

Having a commitment to this mission means having a vision of what the health care system of the future needs to be. The system of the future certainly will always include acute care nursing. Clearly we have the same mandate as do the physicians—we must step back a bit from the acute care bias and prepare ourselves and our graduates for community-based care systems. The National League for Nursing has been quite explicit in its 1993 position paper, "A Vision for Nursing Education," in recommending a "shift in emphasis for all programs to . . . a community-based, community-focused health care system." This does not mean that we can stop assuring that our graduates have a sound base in acute care practice. If we are to meet the demand for the functions of the ACNP, however we envision the exact role, this practice must have a firm foundation. We cannot give up our work to develop the science of acute care nursing. Hospitals, acute illness, and patients who are desperately, acutely ill will always exist and they will need advanced practice nurses as much as ever in the system of the future.

To the extent that we want our acute care facilities of the future to be places in which basic graduates can practice their profession at the level we teach, we need to have knowledgeable managers, staff development educators, and CNSs. Acute care nurse practitioners will be providing just a fraction of all of the care that a patient receives. We will not have accomplished much if we do not ensure that we have other expert nurses in the system to maintain a professional practice environment, to teach and support the nurse at the bedside, to assume responsibility for sophisticated clinical nursing programs, to monitor and evaluate the standard of nursing care. It would be a dreadful mistake to put all of our resources into ACNP programs, just as it would be a mistake to ignore the demand.

We believe that schools have a role in directing change, not just responding to it. We must not make the mistake hospitals have made in thinking we all have to do everything and we can not possibly reach cooperative agreements with our colleagues at other institutions. It is entirely possible to reach agreements that some schools would retain their management programs, others their education track, and others the CNS tracks. We will need to be creative in designing core curricula that allow us to graduate small classes in these specialties without exorbitant expense. Further, we must continue to explore alternative teaching modalities, such as long-distance learning modules, so that we can fulfill our mission of helping steer health care reform.

WORK TO BE DONE

Although the main purpose of this chapter has been to serve as a general introduction for the rest of this book, we also wish to alert the reader from the outset that there is much work still to be done in establishing the role of ACNP and assuring its continued development. This work lies in three areas—practice, education, and the profession.

Practice

In the practice arena, we will have to continue to work on prescriptive authority. Most states now have some form of prescriptive authority for advanced practice nurses (APNs), although this is an *independent* authority in only 22 states (Pearson, 1993). Even in those states progressive enough to have independence, prescriptive authority in hospitals, rather than outpatient settings, is still very new. We cannot afford to become complacent anywhere regarding this issue; the debate about prescriptive authority is not over.

Resolving the prescriptive authority question is part of the larger issue of keeping our state nurse practice acts updated as needed to reflect the changing scope of practice. Most states have some form of advanced practice language in their laws, but these also will need continued attention.

The third practice area for future work concerns the problem of evaluation. We have much work to do in this area and not a great deal of experience. It is especially important for new roles, or for any role that generates as much ambivalence, if not outright opposition, that we provide data regarding effectiveness. Indicators of effectiveness and efficiency might include such things as work load, competencies achieved and maintained, standard performance evaluations, and patient outcome data such as length of stay reports or morbidity data. Our students have to be prepared to begin their data collection the moment they begin their new role; consequently, we should be including this content in their graduate programs.

Education

In the area of education the most immediate need, as we respond to the demand for ACNP programs, is to give some thought to how we can help the faculty become prepared to teach these subjects. The most obvious approaches are either to contract with faculty of one of the schools that has some experience with ACNPs to come on site to provide concentrated course work for the faculty, or to send selected faculty members to the site of other programs. This investment in formal preparation for the faculty not only makes sense in terms of giving the faculty member a good basis for teaching, but it also may make it possible for the acute care faculty to develop a clinical practice of their own. They then may be eligible to join faculty practice plans, something that is generally difficult to arrange in acute care.

The length of the educational program for ACNPs is a growing issue. As is well known, there was a marked effort in the early 1980s to shorten graduate programs and to accommodate part-time students, coinciding with the reduction in federal support of graduate students and the growing need for our students to remain employed. This change makes perfect sense in terms of the financial realities of the times. However, it is becoming increasingly difficult to address the need to socialize students into new and controversial roles on a part-time basis, and equally difficult to teach the needed content and allow time to assimilate the content in just 35 to 40 semester credits. This is a real conundrum and one that will require some very careful consideration over the next few years.

Evaluation is, of course, another aspect of educational planning that must be addressed. One advantage of thinking about how we should evaluate the ACNP educational program before it is initiated is that evaluation can be built in from the outset. Usually these programs begin on a fairly small scale and it would be helpful to follow the graduates and obtain both their evaluation of their education's strengths and weaknesses and some feedback from facilities employing them.

Profession

The final area to think about in terms of future agendas is a familiar one to the nursing profession. Our old ambivalence about differentiated practice is about to become reactivated on an even more complex and urgent level. It seems that it can only become more paradoxical to call many individuals by the same name, to grant the same basic licensure, when the scope of practice and depth of responsibilities of these professionals are growing ever more disparate. We may not be any more ready, as a profession, to address this issue now than we were 10 or 15 years ago, but the continued expansion of advanced practice roles will force us to think about this again.

CONCLUSION

In closing, it surely can be said that "it's not like the old days." While the role of the ACNP is not a panacea for all the ills of the acute care system, it is a most hopeful and exciting development and a real compliment to the demonstrated competence of the NPs and CNSs who have come before us. The three missions described here—adding to the work force to meet market demand, preparing advanced practitioners of the nursing profession, and contributing to the overall design of the health care system—are individually necessary and jointly sufficient. That is, an ACNP educational program or practice model that grows from a limited vision of only one mission will be inadequate to our social responsibility. Aiming at all of these joint missions and focusing our efforts on the work still to be done will provide the direction for the continued evolution of this role in a way that benefits our consumers, our professional peers, and ourselves.

REFERENCES

American Association of Critical Care Nurses & American Nurses Association. (1995). *Scope of practice for the acute care nurse practitioner and the standards of clinical practice for the acute care nurse practitioner.* Washington, DC, American Nurses Association.

American Nurses Association. (1995). *A social policy statement (revised).* Washington, DC: Author.

Clochesy, J. M., Daly, B. J., Idemoto, B. K., Steel, J., & Fitzpatrick, J. J. (1994). Preparing Advanced Practice Nurses for acute care. *Amer Journal of Critical Care, 3*(4), 255–258.

Dale, J. C. (1991). New role for PNPs in an inpatient setting. *Journal of Pediatric Health Care, 5*(6), 336.

Goksel, D., Harrison, C. J., Morrison, R. E., & Miller, S. T. (1993). Description of a nurse practitioner inpatient service in a public teaching hospital. *Journal of General Internal Medicine, 8,* 29–30.

Keane, A., & Richmond, T. (1993). Tertiary care nurse practitioners. *Image, 25*(4), 281–284.

National League for Nursing. (1993). *A vision for nursing education.* New York: Author.

Pearson, L. J. (1993). 1992–93 update: How each state stands on legislative issues affecting advanced nursing practice. *Nurse Practitioner, 18*(1), 23–38.

Shah, H. S., Sullivan, D. T., Lattanzio, J., & Bruttomesso, K. M. (1993). Preparing acute care nurse practitioners at the University of Connecticut. *AACN Clinical Issues, 4*(4), 625–629.

Weinberg, R. M., Liljestrand, J. S., & Moore, S. (1983). Inpatient management by a nurse practitioner: Effectiveness in a rehabilitation setting. *Archives of Physical Medicine and Rehabilitation, 64,* 588–590.

Chapter 2

DEVELOPMENT OF THE ACUTE CARE NURSE PRACTITIONER ROLE: QUESTIONS, OPINIONS, CONSENSUS

Jean E. Steel, PhD, RN, FAAN

The establishment, development, and growth of the nurse practitioner role has been a relatively brief part of nursing's history, but this role has had a major impact on the advancement of nursing and the improvement of health care services. These last 25 years have been unprecedented in the application of knowledge to practice, the development of collaborative models of health care, and the explosion of the legal regulation of advanced practice. In fact, the development of the term "advanced practice" itself stems from the complexities and wide variation among roles for nurses with graduate preparation and the need to establish one label that denotes a level of practice applicable within all specialties.

Just as current social and political trends and forces are shaped by the events of the past, the emergence of the ACNP role has been directly influenced by the way in which its predecessor, the primary care nurse practitioner role, was created and grew. The purpose of this chapter is to review salient points in the history of the nurse practitioner movement, highlighting questions and issues that have been particularly significant or suggest important parallels with the acute care role. This perspective will be used to suggest areas for discussion and further consideration by those in the profession who will shape the continued evolution of the ACNP.

HISTORICAL SYNOPSIS

Origins and Early Stages

The need to develop a new area of expansion in nursing occurred because of a changing social environment. Large sectors of the population had no access to care. Further, the public was seeking new alternatives to disease care and welcomed the nursing approach that included health promotion and improved life styles. In addition, consistent with social initiatives in other areas, consumers were also seeking a choice in their provider. While both nurses and physicians could provide equal services for a selected cluster of conditions, the overlap of activities offered the promise of a larger provider network.

It is important to note that the generic term "nurse practitioner" (NP) in the early stages described the nurse providing care in ambulatory settings. No programs were preparing NPs to practice in the acute care setting until the early 1990s. Thus the term nurse practitioner was assumed to refer only to persons practicing outside of the acute care hospital. The curricula and clinical practice of the NP were designed exclusively for ambulatory settings and the graduate was expected to be an employee of an outpatient facility, including clinics, private offices, health maintenance organizations, etc. In some cases, the NP established private practices, either alone or in partnership with others.

Ford and Silver are credited with the development of the original NP program, which prepared nurses to deliver pediatric care in rural Colorado in 1965 (Ford & Silver, 1967). The first projects in academic settings were interested in recruiting public health nurses who held a baccalaureate degree in nursing and were eligible for graduate admission at the University of Colorado (Ford & Silver, 1967). Other programs quickly emerged throughout the country, located in a variety of settings, including universities and hospitals. The establishment of the pediatric NP was closely followed by programs focused on care of the adult, family, and older client. The movement gained further momentum as the programs of short duration in continuing education moved into graduate study in Schools of Nursing. By 1994, most programs were located in graduate programs, taught by nursing school faculty.

Extensive evaluation of the NP role and outcomes associated with NP care came next. By 1978, over 600 articles and studies on the effectiveness of the NP had been published (Winterton, 1978). Early literature presented the experiences of faculty, students, and programs. By the early 1970s, the literature was describing the competence of the practitioner in assuming responsibility for assessment and management of health problems. Since then the literature has continued to validate the quality of care provided by NPs and has reported extensive consumer satisfaction data.

More recently, discussions have focused on the challenges related to education, work in different clinical settings, research, and the administration of NP practices. One journal was established to provide service to NPs and their practice, *The Nurse Practitioner: American Journal of Primary Health Care*, while other journals, such as the *American Journal of Nursing*, have developed special features intended to target NPs.

Many studies have been conducted to examine the role, the nurse, the practice and the outcomes of care. The work of Lewis and Resnick (1967), Yankhauer, Tripp, Andrews, and Connelly (1974), Spitzer et al. (1974), and Sultz, Soelenzy, Matthews, and Kinyon (1980) was seminal in the early years. Official organizations conducted studies which further verified the effectiveness of the NP, including the Office of Technology (1986) and the American Nurses Association (ANA) (Brown and Grimes 1993). These studies have been important in the gradual acceptance of the role of the NP by the wider health care community.

Of particular relevance, the Brown and Grimes (1993) meta-analysis of 38 controlled studies compared NPs and physicians in terms of processes of care, clinical outcomes and the cost-effectiveness of resource utilization. The analysis examined variables such as rates of drug prescription, number of visits per patient, average spending on laboratory tests, mortality rates, and incidence of complications of birth. This study yielded the significant finding that advanced practice nurses (APNs) had patient care outcomes equivalent to or somewhat better than those of physicians. This finding was consistent with the summary of the Office of Technology Assessment (1986).

Crucial to the acceptance of the NP role has been the early efforts to work collaboratively with representatives of organized medicine. In the early 1970s, the National Joint Practice Commission (NJPC) was founded as a collaborative venture by the American Nurses Association and the American Medical Association. The emerging role of NP was discussed and examined, and extensive literature was created that described the value of a collaborative effort between nursing and medicine. Professional issues and overlapping responsibilities were examined and position papers were developed. The NJPC elevated the concept of collaboration between medicine and nursing to new heights and primed both disciplines to establish new liaisons (Steel, 1986).

Initial Conflict

Throughout the 1970s and early 1980s, NP education was based in continuing education programs. The faculty of these early programs were predominantly physicians. This undoubtedly contributed to a divisiveness within the profession of nursing between NPs, those supporting this emerging role, and nurses who opposed this form of advanced practice. Those who had little understanding of the genesis of the NP's work claimed that the role was essentially a physician's assistant role and insisted that the NP was working outside of the domain of nursing.

The insistence that the NP role was outside of the domain of nursing primarily stemmed from the fact that it incorporated new skills and delegated to the nurse functions previously in the domain of medicine. Nurse practitioner skills were often understood as consisting solely of history taking and physical examination. However, from the outset, these skills have represented only a small portion of the work of the NP and nurses at all levels have always been expected to provide assessment and management as part of their practice. The primary function of the nurse did not change with the establishment of the NP role. Indeed, the fundamental responsibility of the professional nurse today, regardless of level, continues to be health maintenance, disease prevention, and care of clients in sickness and health. Simply stated, "nursing is the diagnosis and treatment of human responses to actual or potential health problems"(ANA, 1980, p.9).

Conflict within the profession continued throughout the early development of the NP role. Comparisons and contrasts with the work of the clinical nurse specialist (CNS) raised many debates and further splintered the evolution of advanced practice. Partly in response to this internal competition, NPs felt the need to establish their own professional organizations to provide an exclusive voice to legislators and to public regulators. Faculty in Schools of Nursing were fervently divided as to where the education of the NP belonged and certifying agencies were delayed in the development of a credential for the NP. Members of Boards of Nursing who were asked to regulate the work of the NP appeared beset by doubts and differences in opinions.

Partial resolution of these conflicts occurred by the end of the 1970s with the belief that the educational preparation of the NP was suited for graduate study in Schools of Nursing. One of the stimuli for this resolution was that public funding required the program to reside in a graduate program in nursing, granting a master's degree. Advanced practice, based on nursing theory and linked with outcomes demonstrated through research, justified the expansion of nursing's domain, with greater emphasis being placed on a specialty body of knowledge and less on the NP role. As more and more graduates emerged from programs, new practice sites were found and NPs moved into a host of new settings and specialties. This expansion then afforded more nurses and physicians first-hand experience working with NPs and helped to educate others about the contributions NPs could make to the care of patients.

CURRENT STATUS OF THE NURSE PRACTITIONER

By the end of 1992, there were more than 42,000 nurses prepared as NPs and employed in nursing (Moses, 1992). This figure represents approximately one third of all nurses in advanced practice. Nurse practitioners, consistent with the requirements of advanced practice, are prepared at the graduate level with a master's degree in nursing. Course work includes nursing systems, research, theory, assessment and management, pharmacology, behavioral counseling, pathophysiology, clinical reasoning, and a variety of subspecialty topics (see chapter 4 for further details on curricula). Nurse practitioners provide care within the domain of their expertise. Using expert assessment techniques and sound principles of clinical decision making, they act as case managers, direct care providers, educators and consultants. In at least 44 state jurisdictions across the country, NPs have some form of prescriptive authority (Pearson, 1995). They use a variety of treatment modalities, not limited to medicines alone, to prevent illness and treat disease.

Educational programs that prepare NPs have developed throughout the country, and virtually every school of nursing offering a master's degree has added an NP program track recently. As the demand for the role of case manager has grown and as economic pressures have created more interest in alternative primary health care providers, schools have rushed to develope programs to attract students, even though they may not employ NPs on their regular faculty. The rapidity of the growth of NP programs has led to concern about the quality of educational programs, particularly in regard to the qualifications of faculty. The uniqueness and value of a program lie in the experience and expertise of the faculty members as NPs themselves, developed through classroom study, precepted clinical placements and experience as graduate nurse practitioners.

Unresolved Issues and Challenges

Despite the important strides that have been made in gaining recognition of the contribution of NPs in the health care arena, several significant roadblocks remain. Direct reimbursement for services rendered by an NP has been slow and inconsistent in the implementation of public law. In parts of the country, private insurers pay for care provided by an NP, while in other locations, they deny payment to nurses. Several federal initiatives have been created to stimulate reimbursement but they have had varying success in different states (Mittelstadt, 1993). Some reimbursement systems permit a percent reduction when the services are provided by an NP. A variety of efforts over the years have failed to convince policy makers of the need for "equal pay for equal work."

For NPs to evolve as independent professionals, separate from and not under the authority of medicine, lobbying and strengthening of the recognition of nursing's contribution among professional colleagues will have to continue. Although some of the responsibilities of advanced practice nurses have been delegated to them by physicians, these activities do not lie solely and permanently within the domain of medicine and thus do not require medical supervision. Clearly, if a procedure or skill is taught by nursing faculty as part of a nursing curriculum, and the practitioner has repeated opportunities to carry out the activity under established practice guidelines or protocols, that activity must belong to nursing. Continued study, consensus and development of the ownership of once delegated activities will need continual examination and research.

The formal barriers to advanced nursing practice have been eloquently discussed by Safreit (1992). It is important to recognize that, despite the existence of narrow and specific advanced nurse practice acts in some states, the professional scope of practice does not vary from state to state. The American Nurses Association has developed a scope of practice description and standards of practice for nurse practitioners; these position papers apply to all nurse practitioners. Although some states have sought amendments to their practice acts to include the NP (and usually the clinical nurse specialist, nurse midwife, and nurse anesthetist), as the role and education of the nurse has constantly changed, these amendments have had the effect of overregulating advanced practice (Hadley, 1989). As a result, there may be less freedom to advance the profession in keeping with society's changing needs. This is a danger that will apply to all advanced practice roles in the future.

EVOLUTION OF ACUTE CARE NURSE PRACTITIONERS

Setting the Stage

In 1990, the ACNP emerged as one solution to the changing conditions in acute care environments. The turbulent health care environment produced fragmented delivery systems which were staggering under the increased demands for care. Access to care, short hospital stays, the aging population and an increase in chronic conditions all contributed to the stress felt by acute care settings. Professional resources prepared to meet increased demand and cost were limited and delegation of activities was prevalent. Quality of care was jeopardized in many locations and personnel were stretched to meet greater patient needs without additional resources. Managed care was seen as a method of assuring integration and coordination of needed care and advocacy for patients and their families (Bower, 1992). It became clear that there was a need to develop an ACNP role to "respond to patients" needs across the full continuum of acute care services (ANA, 1995, p. 10).

Complimenting the ACNP role is the CNS. Because both roles fit within the context of advanced nursing practice, there are similarities in their functions. There is some agreement that the roles have merged in many settings and are no longer distinguishable in the care that is provided. Previously, the NP was seen only as an expert in history-taking and physical examination, devoting the majority of his/her time to direct patient care. Clinical Nurse Specialists also provided some direct care, but included consultation, research, and education as part of their work. Today, both roles include all of these activities, although to differing degrees or with varying emphasis on different aspects (Elder & Bullough, 1990; Fenton & Brykczynski, 1993; Lieber, 1993; Steel, 1994).

Coincidentally, the merger of roles is predictable as one of the results of needed health care reform. The measure of achievement in the health care economy is in direct relationship to the provision of patient services. If APNs do not provide patient care services, their inclusion on the clinical staff may be in serious jeopardy. This economic reality has encouraged both the development of the ACNP role as a new provider of care and, in some settings, a shift in the focus of CNSs.

To fully understand the evolution of a role for NPs in care of persons experiencing an acute illness, it may be helpful to consider the conceptual basis of all advanced practice. Nursing, as an applied science, selects and applies theories from the existing sciences to understand and treat those conditions within the domain of nursing. Because of the monumental explosion of technology and scientific knowledge over the past decade, nursing specialists have rapidly expanded their domain to provide specialty nursing care. Specialists who have received advanced preparation at the graduate level are able to focus their efforts on a particular aspect of clinical nursing, test applications of newly available theories to conditions germane to clinical care, translate theory applications into nursing approaches and assist in encouraging and speeding the flow of new knowledge into basic education and generalized nursing practice (ANA, 1980).

The term "advanced nursing practice" refers to the activities of nurses who have acquired knowledge and practice in specialty areas that further permit expansion and advancement of the profession. Specialization focuses on a part of the practice of nursing. Expansion refers to the acquisition of new practice skills. Advancement of the professional nurse and of the profession itself occurs as a result of both specialization and expansion (ANA, 1995).

The emphasis in this process of advancement is on the body of knowledge, not the role that one takes in the work setting. Thus, the relevant body of knowledge and specialization in this instance is acute and critical care. Through this specialization and expansion of activities, the work of the ACNP advances the profession.

Over the years, nurses in acute care settings have been refining skills, applying new knowledge and assuming increasing responsibility for care. Patients have recovered because of the nearness and constancy of the nurse. In some cases, the nurse in the acute care setting has been given added authority along with responsibility, but this has often been couched in what Stein refers to as "the doctor-nurse game" or the "strange way nurses recommend to physicians" (Stein, 1967). This "transactional neurosis" permits the doctor to give the order for treatment, based on the nurse's recommendation. In fact, it gives authority to the physician for "orders" but it is based on the nurse's observation, knowledge, and specific recommendation. Now, with the advent of the ACNP role, the authority to carry out the patient's care is in the domain of nursing. As with development of the primary care NP, the laws permitting this authority will have to change to reflect actual practice.

Preliminary Issues

The definition of the ACNP role is simply to "provide advanced nursing care across the continuum of acute care services to patients who are acutely and critically ill" (ANA, 1995, p. 11). The NP is part of a team of professionals, collaborating to provide needed care. The ACNP complements the other team members and demonstrates expertise in a specialty focus of nursing care.

In 1995, the Scope of Practice was written by the American Nurses Association and the American Association of Critical Care Nurses (ANA, 1995) working in collaboration with each other. This document describes the parameters of the role and contains the standards for clinical practice and professional performance. As the role evolves, these standards of performance will be refined as appropriate. Revisions are expected as practitioners discover new techniques, apply new knowledge and respond to society's ever changing needs.

The relationship of the ACNP to medicine is a strategic one, requiring sincere collaborative efforts in the implementation of the early programs. Physicians' authority to perform certain procedures will be delegated to the ACNP through education and practice. The original clinical preceptors therefore will be physicians in the clinical arena. As APNs graduate into the role of the ACNP, they will assume responsibility for clinical preceptorships with new graduate nursing students.

Collaborative efforts with medicine go beyond program development and are necessary in the actual delivery of care. Because many of the new procedures are delegated from medicine to nursing, medical supervision (in the clinical area) for these procedures will be exercised for some time to come. Gradually, however, these activities will fall within the domain of nursing's legal and professional scope. It is imperative that the relationship between nurse and physician continue as a collaborative, not competitive or supervisory, one. The focus must be on the patient/family and their needs and not on the role of the provider. That is, the identification of patient and family needs should determine who the dominant provider of that care will be.

Acute care nurse practitioners will also need to be alert to collaborative relationships with others, most especially nurse colleagues. Just as the NP is discovering new roles, these roles will need interpretation to others. Avoiding competition will enhance the care of patients and further advance the profession. Because nursing is a dynamic rather than static profession, the boundaries expand outward. "As new needs and demands impinge upon nursing . . . the defining characteristics of scope begin to change" (ANA,1980, p. 16). In the early development of roles, all professionals deal with ambiguity. The ability to live with ambiguity and feel professionally sound is a challenge to ACNPs.

Professional Resolution

Many questions arise with the establishment of a new role. These include issues related to how nurses are educated, the focus of nursing research, how students are socialized and what credentialing is used as the method of public accountability.

Implications for Educators

The trumpet call of health care reform is a call to how access and care should be organized, costed and distributed. The development of the ACNP permits acute care educators to take bold new steps in their curriculum development (Clochesy, Daly, Idemoto, Steel, & Fitzpatrick, 1994). Schools of nursing have responded to real needs in the clinical setting, needs expressed by administrators and patients. Curricula have been revitalized and refocused on specialty knowledge and clinical expertise. Knowledge relevant to the care of conditions has been reintroduced and strengthened through the application of appropriate sciences.

The faculty member's responsibility is to guide the graduate student through the educational experience, acting as a role model and demonstrating competence in the problems germane to the specialty area (ANA, 1980). This expectation permits and encourages nursing faculty to fulfill their role as teacher and collaborator with others in the field. When possible, the faculty compliment of university programs will be strengthened with the addition of acute care nurse practitioners, perhaps as clinical associates.

The breadth of experience and the creative wisdom of this team of faculty will result in a rich experience for students and will prepare experts for the clinical field. The challenge is to assure quality and substance in the NP education (Booth, 1995). Clochesy and Daly (chapter 4) have identified some of the central issues to be addressed by faculty in the curricular design phase of new ACNP programs.

In preparing the ACNP, the traditional rotation in a clinical practicum may not be appropriate for the mastery of skills and application of knowledge. A variety of models are being tested as to how the practicum requirement can be achieved in acute settings with the rapid turnover of patients. (For a more detailed discussion see chapter 5.)

One of the central challenges in education of ACNPs is the problem of providing a meaningful clinical experience in the usual 12 to 16-hour day. It is difficult to "practice" being a case manager one or two days a week. An example of innovations that are being tried is the "executive" model. This practicum, which fulfills the total clinical hours requirement, is planned for one full semester of full time (40 hours per week) study. This 600-hour experience is equivalent to the traditional part-time experiences that are spread out over several semesters. This arrangement permits the student to synthesize theory and clinical findings, use bioethical decision making, and practice as a case manager in a precepted environment. Also, mastery of advanced therapeutics, both pharmacological and nonpharmacological, is expected at the end of this practicum.

The advantages of an executive practicum must be weighed against possible disadvantages. Clearly, one of these disadvantages is the time commitment required of students who usually are enrolled in a part-time status. In addition, it is difficult to plan this type of practicum if the student is expected to attend core courses during this semester. Whatever model is chosen and tested, educators and clinical faculty will need to collaborate in designing a practicum to meet student need and patient care expectations.

How do we socialize the ACNP?

As the curriculum changes to focus on the preparation of the ACNP, proportionately more of the education may take place in the clinical setting. Mentoring by university faculty in collaboration with clinically based experts will enrich the experience for students.

Nonetheless, it is imperative that ACNPs receive the core knowledge for all graduate nurse students. Being with other students in advanced practice permits open dialogue, inquiry and understanding. The need for in-depth clinical experience in addition to the same theory and research requirements of other graduate students may have implications for the length of ACNP programs. Further experience is needed to evaluate this.

Credentialing of the ACNP

Credentialing includes licensure, certification and accreditation. The ACNP enters the field, as do all nurses, through the designation of registered nurse (RN); eligibility for advanced practice privileges, such as prescriptive authority and the right to use a specific title then rests on meeting the additional requirements of the state in which he or she practices. At present, there is no specific language that singularly designates the ACNP. This is not necessarily problematic and, in fact, may permit the evolution of the role to rapidly expand, rather than prematurely close, the boundaries for responsibility and authority.

The establishment of a scope of practice and standards of clinical performance are the first steps toward a formal method of certification. The ANA and AACN have initiated a joint-certification offering, available to graduates of a master's program preparing specialists in acute care. This certification will permit the individual nurse to be recognized by state statutes requiring certification by a national credentialing body and to practice within the boundaries of advanced practice in that jurisdiction. In some states, the certified ACNP will receive prescriptive authority from the state board of registration.

Although professional certification was originally a voluntary achievement and not intended to regulate entry into the practice, many state laws require certification to practice. Thus, the eligibility to sit for an NP certification does not include minimum years of practice. Standards and policies that regulate the practice of all NPs in the future will be similar. This is imperative for the public's understanding of the specialist. Further, a registry of appropriately credentialled specialists should be established as a form of designation. This may prevent the double licensing of the nurse in advanced practice.

CONCLUSION

The history of the primary care NP's development from the late 1960s onward is a reference for the development of the ACNP. Some mysteries and pitfalls have been avoided or short-circuited. The similarities in development are profound. The value of considering similar patterns of evolution lies in the insights to be gained and the preparedness that can come from studying any history of events. There is much to be learned from those who have gone before us.

The continuing evolution of professional nursing is evident in the role of the ACNP. The development and implementation of this role has rapidly descended on nurse clinicians, educators, administrators, and practitioners. It has evolved because of the need to establish the nurse as a patient care manager and a provider of quality health care. This role offers a new venue for the contributions of acute and critical care nurses, expanding the boundaries and responsibilities of nursing practice. The need for reform in health care, the changing mix of hospital providers, and the enthusiasm of nursing leaders in the development of this role, all these offer opportunities to the profession, opportunities that are both controversial, inspiring, and hopeful.

REFERENCES

American Nurses Association. (1980). *Nursing: A social policy statement.* Kansas City, MO: American Nurses Association.

American Nurses Association. (1995). Nursing; A social policy statement; revised. Washington, DC: American Nurses Association.

American Nurses Association. (1995). *Standards of clinical practice and scope of practice for the Acute Care Nurse Practitioner.* Washington, DC: American Nurses Association and American Association of Critical Care Nurses.

Booth, R. (1995). Leadership challenges for nurse practitioner faculty. *Nurse Practitioner, 20*:4(April 1995), 52–58.

Bower, K. A. (1993). *Case management by nurses.* American Nurse Association, Washington, DC: The American Nurses Association.

Brown, S. A., & Grimes, D. E. (1993). *A meta-analysis of process of care, clinical outcomes and cost-effectiveness of nurses in primary care roles; nurse practitioners and certified nurse midwives.* Prepared for the ANA Division of Health Policy. Washington, DC: American Nurses Association.

Clochesy J., Daly, B., Idemoto, B., Steel, J., & Fitzpatrick, J. (1994). Preparing advanced practice nurses for acute care. *American Journal of Critical Care, 4,* 255–258.

Elder R. G., & Bullough, B. (1990). Nurse practitioners and clinical nurse specialists; are the roles merging? *Clinical Nurse Specialist, 4*(2), 78–84.

Fenton, M. V., & Brykczynski, K. A. (1993). Qualitative distinctions and similarities in the practice of clinical nurse specialists and nurse practitioners. *Journal of Professional Nursing, 9*(6), 313–326.

Ford, L., & Silver, H. (1967). The expanded role of the nurse in child care. *Nursing Outlook, 15* (September), 43–45.

Hadley, E. H. (1989). Nurses and prescriptive authority; A legal and economic analysis. *American Journal of Law and Medicine, XV*(Nos 2–3), 245–299.

Lewis, C., & Resnick, B. (1967). Nurses clinics and progressive ambulatory patient care. *New England Journal of Medicine, 277,* 1236–1241.

Lieber, M. T. (1993). Looking toward an NP/CNS merger by the year 2010 (Letter to the editor). *Nurse Practitioner, 18*(4a), 15, 19, 43.

Mittelstadt, P. C. (1993). Federal reimbursement of advanced practice nurses' services empowers the profession. *Nurse Practitioner, 18*(1), 43–49.

Moses, E. (1992). *The Registered nurse population; Findings from the national sample survey of registered nurses,* March 1992. Washington, DC: U.S. Department of Health and Human Services, Division of Nursing.

Office of Technology. (1986). *Nurse practitioners, physician assistants, and certified midwives; a policy analysis.* Health Technology Case Study

#37. Office of Technology Assessment, Congress of the United States, Washington, DC.

Pearson, L. (1995). Annual update; how each state stands on legislative issues affecting advanced nursing practice. *Nurse Practitioner, 20*(1), 13–51.

Safriet, B. (1992). Health care dollars and regulatory sense; the role of advanced practice nursing. *Yale Journal of Regulation, 9,* 417–488.

Spitzer, W. A., Sacket D. L., Sibley, J. C., Roberts, R. S., Gent, M., Kergin, D. J., Hackett, B. C., & Olynich, A. (1974). The Burlington Randomized Trial of the nurse practitioner. *New England Journal of Medicine, 290,* 251–256.

Steel, J. E. (1986). *Issues in Collaborative Practice.* Grune and Stratton, Orlando, FL.

Steel, J. E. (1994). Advanced nursing practice. *AACN Clinical Issues in Critical Care Nursing, 5*(1), 71–76.

Stein, L. (1967). The doctor-nurse game. *Archires of General Psychiatry, 16,* 699–703.

Sultz, H., Soelenzy, M., Matthews, J., & Kinyon, L. (1980). Longitudinal study of nurse practitioners; phase I-III. DPH Publication, No. HRA 80-2. Hyattsville, MD.

Winterton, M. E. (1978). Evaluation of nurse practitioner effectiveness; an overview of the literature. *Evaluation and the Health Professions, 1*(1), 69–81.

Yankhauer, A., Tripp, S., Andrews, P., & Connelly, J. (1974). The outcomes and service impact of a pediatric nurse practitioner training program; nurse practitioner training outcomes. *American Journal of Public Health, 62,* 347–353.

Chapter 3

INFLUENCE OF THE HEALTH CARE ENVIRONMENT

Barbara J. Daly, PhD, RN, FAAN
Carol Genet, MSN, RN, CS

Health care takes place in an environment of change. This has always been true because of the commitment of health care professionals to strive for improvements in our ability to treat and prevent illness and disease. In the past, the focus of our efforts has been on discovering and testing interventions and, for nurses, understanding human response to illness. This orientation has been tremendously successful in enabling us to cure an increasing number of diseases and reduce the effects of illness. However, at the same time, our lack of attention to the system itself has resulted in inefficiencies, out-of-control spending, and barriers to use by all but the most sophisticated consumers.

No one associated with acute care today can be unaware of the aggressive attempts to change this situation. Driven primarily by economic forces, virtually all hospitals are undergoing restructuring, reorganization, and redesign. It is this feature of acute care that has created the need for a new role, the acute care nurse practitioner

(ACNP). The purpose of this chapter is to provide a discussion of the specific forces in the health care environment that created this demand and to evaluate the way in which these forces have contributed to the ACNP role development.

MODERN TERTIARY CARE

The characteristics of the modern acute care facility that led to these needs for a new kind of practitioner are well known. Today's hospital is more "user unfriendly" than ever before, due in large part to the increasing orientation toward narrow specialties and impressive use of sophisticated technologies. These characteristics, while successful in producing significant advances in our ability to treat specific organ dysfunctions, have also led to significant increases in cost. The resulting mandate to address out-of-control spending patterns has been associated with aggressive reductions in some areas of hospital spending and changes in patterns of service provision.

The modern hospital of today is a dual-function institution. It exists for at least two purposes: care of acutely ill persons and the education of physicians. The level, type, and organization of services reflects this dual purpose and leads directly to both increased cost and greater burdens on patients faced with negotiating a complex bureaucracy. This is particularly problematic for our most vulnerable patients, the elderly and chronically ill, who are poorly equipped to compensate for the inefficiencies of a system designed around learning needs of students rather than care needs of patients.

Trends in the Profession of Medicine

The profession of medicine is characterized today by both a general oversupply of physicians and an excess of specialists over generalists. Factors which have contributed to this pattern include the increased fees and general earning power of specialists, the increased prestige accorded to specialists, and a reimbursement scheme that has favored performance of technologic procedures over such activities

TABLE 3.1   Specialization Among U.S. Physicians

GROUP	1970 (millions)	1990 (millions)	% Increase
U.S. population	203,212	248,710	22
Professional active MDs	310,845	547,310	76
Residents + Interns	45,840	81,664	78
Office-based Practices			
General/Family	50,816	57,571	13
General Surgery	18,068	24,498	35
Orthopedic Surgery	6,533	14,187	117
Anesthesiology	7,369	17,789	141
Internal Medicine	22,950	57,799	152
Cardiovascular	3,882	10,670	175
Pulmonary	785	3,659	366
Gastroenterology	1,112	5,200	368
Neurology	1,192	5,587	369
Diagnostic Radiology	896	9,806	994

Source: *Health United States, 1992.* Hyattsville, MD: Department of Health and Human Services, National Center for Health Statistics. DHHS Pub. No. (PHS) 93-1232, p. 144.

as health promotion and patient education (Petersdorf, 1993; Wennberg, Goodman, Nease, & Keller, 1993).

As shown in Table 3.1, there has been a 76% increase in the number of professionally active physicians and a 78% increase in the number of interns and residents in nonfederal hospitals over the past 20 years. During this same period the population in the United States increased only 22%. The largest increases, ranging from 366 to 994%, were in the specialties of diagnostic radiology, neurology, gastroenterology, and pulmonary medicine, while the number of physicians in general medicine/family practice increased only 13% (Health United States, 1992, 1993).

While the number of physicians in internal medicine has continued to grow, it has been noted for some time that the interest in internal medicine programs has declined compared to past decades.

Surveys of medical students have shown that careers in internal medicine are perceived as more stressful and demanding of time and less personally satisfying and financially rewarding than the careers of specialists (Babbott, Levey, Weaver, & Killian, 1991; Schwartz, Linzer, Babbott, Divine, & Broadhead, 1991). Although not specifically mentioned in these reports, the uncertainty regarding the financial situation may stem from worries about the ability to repay educational loans.

The increasing use of specialists is problematic for several reasons. First, it increases costs. The referral and subsequent treatment by a specialist represents two provider visits (first to the generalist, then to the specialist) and the specialist is more likely to use sophisticated and expensive diagnostic and treatment modalities. The factor responsible for the largest percentage of annual increase in health care costs in the past, after general price inflation, has been the increase in the intensity and volume of health services (see Figure 3.1). This

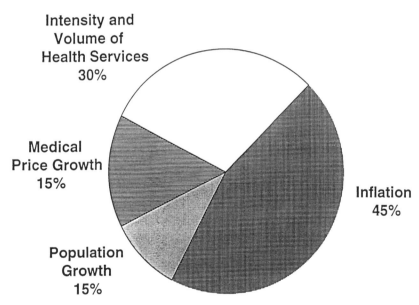

FIGURE 3.1 Factors contributing to increased spending, 1989–1990.

Source: Committee on Ways and Means, U.S. House of Representatives. (1991). *Health care resource book.* Washington, DC: U.S. Government Printing Office.

reflects both the overuse of services, compared to other countries, and the propensity to use more costly services, including those of specialists.

In addition to increasing the cost of care, the overuse of specialists has contributed to the complexity and fragmentation of acute care. Although the concept of quality of care is obviously multifaceted, there is general agreement that persons experiencing a crisis of an acute illness, as well as those struggling to manage chronic conditions, benefit from a stable, intimate relationship with a single provider who knows them and can serve as their advocate (Bluestone, 1993; Havre, 1993; Marwick, 1994). Unfortunately, today's world of modern medicine is characterized more by strangeness, distance, diversity, and alienation than by intimacy and familiarity. The average hospitalized patient today, particularly if hospitalized in a tertiary-care center, is probably cared for by a physician he/she met only once before hospitalization and has a separate expert or team responsible for managing each distinct organ dysfunction with little or no coordination of overall care planning. For example, a recent study of chronically critically ill persons reported that patients who remain in intensive care units for several weeks have, on average, eight consulting services contributing to and managing various aspects of care (Daly, Rudy, Thompson, & Happ, 1991). In this context, it is not surprising that patients feel alienated and often perceive their care as disjointed and fragmented.

PATIENT NEEDS

These characteristics are particularly ill suited to meet the needs of acutely ill hospitalized patients because of the characteristics of patients today. The aging of the population in general and the ability to prevent death from acute causes has led to a population of elderly patients with chronic illnesses. The number of elderly in the United States has been steadily growing since the start of this century, and is projected to continue to increase. In 1990 persons over age 65 represented 12.7% of the U.S. population; this age group is expected to represent 21.7% of the population by the year 2050 (U.S. Department of Commerce, Bureau of the Census, 1983).

Probably more germane to this discussion, with increasing age comes an increasing prevalence of chronic diseases and comorbidities. The presence of chronic disease and the overall decreases in physiologic reserves of the elderly complicate the treatment of acute illness and place the individual at greater risk of poor outcomes (Office of Technology Assessment, 1987). For example, the average length of stay for cholecystectomy patients in 1985 (before the widespread use of laparoscopic procedures) was 7.6 days; with multiple diagnoses, the length of stay increased to 11.8 days (Commission on Professional and Hospital Activities, 1986). Among persons over age 65, 38% have some limitation of activity due to a chronic condition (Health United States, 1992, p. 99). Given the increased use of resources necessitated by risk and complexity of care, these patients in particular have a need for someone to coordinate their care and provide comprehensive discharge planning that takes into account their individual social factors. Although these comments seem obvious, a recent study of 900 hospitals revealed that only 9% of elderly patients were discharged with plans for further care (GAO, 1987, quoted in Brooten, 1993).

Cost

Of the myriad of influences on the shape and nature of acute care today, none is more significant than economics. Beginning in the early 1980s, virtually every segment of professional, governmental, and business organizations has focused on strategies designed to reduce the rapidly escalating costs of care in this country. There are three specific strategies that have contributed to the need for the acute care practitioner: reduction in length of stay and redesign aimed at greater efficiency, managed care programs and capitation schemes, and projected decrease in federal support for physician education.

The reductions in average length of stay which began with the implementation of the prospective payment system of Diagnosis Related Groupings (DRGs) are well known. As can be seen in Table 3.2, the number of hospitals, number of admissions/discharges, and the average length of stay began to decrease in 1980 and have continued to the present time. However, the effectiveness of initial strate-

TABLE 3.2   Short-stay Hospital Statistics

Year	Number*	Occupancy Rate	Length of Stay**
1960	5,407	74.7%	7.6 days
1970	5,859	78.0	8.2
1975	5,979	74.8	7.7
1980	5,904	75.4	7.6
1985	5,784	64.8	7.1
1990	5,420	66.8	7.3
1991	5,370	66.1	7.2

*Excludes federal hospitals.
**Excludes psychiatric stays.
Source: Health United States, 1992. Hyattsville, Md.: Department of Health and Human Services, National Center for Health Statistics. DHHS Pub. No. (PHS) 93-1232, pp. 133, 153.

gies of earlier discharges and shifting of procedures to outpatient facilities was short-lived. The slowing of annual increases in total health expenditures lasted only from 1984 to 1988 and has returned to a 0.5–1.0% annual increase since then (see Table 3.3). While these cost reduction efforts of the 1980s and early 1990s have resulted in fewer admissions and shorter stays, thus producing "sicker and quicker" hospitalizations, these initiatives have proven to be inadequate in addressing the underlying causes of excessive spending.

In addition to attempting to lower costs through lowering lengths of stay and providing an incentive for hospitals to reduce spending, cost control has also been attempted through simply restricting the amount reimbursed per admission. An analysis done by the Prospective Payment Assessment Commission has shown that hospital profit margins for Medicare patients in 1985, soon after the initiation of DRGs, was nearly 15%; these margins have decreased and are now negative for many diagnoses (Prospective Payment Assessment Commission, 1994). The inability to obtain reimbursement that at least equals cost for the increasing number of patients using Medi-

TABLE 3.3   Health Expenditures

Year	National Health Expend. (billions)	Health Spending per Capita	Annual % Increase per Capita	Health Spending as % of GNP
1970	$74.4	$346		7.4%
1980	249.1	1,059		8.6
1981	288.6	1,215	14.7%	9.1
1982	323.8	1,349	11.1	9.5
1983	356.1	1,469	8.9	10.2
1984	387.0	1,582	7.6	10.5
1985	420.1	1,700	7.5	10.3
1986	452.3	1,813	6.6	10.7
1987	492.5	1,955	7.8	10.9
1988	544.0	2,139	9.4	11.2
1989	604.1	2,354	10.0	11.6
1990	675.0	2,601	10.5	12.2
1991	751.8	2,868	10.3	13.2
1992	800.0 (est.)			

Source: Committee on Ways Means, U.S. House of Representatives. (1991). *Health care resource book.* Washington, DC: U.S. Government Printing Office, p. 125.

care represents a significant threat to the financial viability of acute care facilities.

The current focus of economic initiatives can be grouped under the term "managed care." This term refers to organizational systems designed to provide, either directly or through contracts with providers, continuous health care services in a cost-effective manner, through the mechanisms of coordination of care, productivity and quality monitoring, and financial incentives to both patients and providers (American Nurses Association, 1995; Koepper, Mess, & Troff, 1995). The growth of the earliest form of managed care, Health Maintenance Organizations (HMOs), as well as the appearance of managed care mandates in virtually every health reform proposal, attests to the belief that only fundamental changes in the way care is organized and provided will have lasting effects on health care spending. Since their inception in the early 1970s, HMO enrollment has increased to more than 44 million members and is pre-dicted to reach almost 150 million enrollees by the year 2000 (see Table 3.4). Capitation, a reimbursement system which prospectively contracts for a set payment per unit of service (usually per enrollee per year), provides a powerful incentive for provider groups and facilities to manage patient care efficiently and to reduce the use of the most expensive interventions. This, in turn, requires coordination of care, aggressive and effective discharge planning which will minimize the occurrence of readmissions, and attention to education and counseling to assist patients in making life style changes to reduce risk of disease.

The third area of cost control which has contributed to the demand for the ACNP role is a decrease in federal support for hospital-based training of interns and residents. Since its inception in 1965, the Medicare program has reimbursed teaching hospitals for a portion of the costs of education of interns and residents. This legislation is based on the recognition that it costs more to care for patients in an academic environment and that teaching hospitals often provide services to the indigent in the form of clinics staffed by residents, as well as a belief that educational support would promote high-quality care for Medicare recipients (Aiken, 1995). Hospitals receive payments under Medicare, referred to as "pass-through" expenses, according to the number of interns and residents and the intern/resident-to-bed ratio. In 1992, these payments totaled $6.6 billion (Johnson, 1994). Coupled with payments to practice plans for patient care services, this represents almost half of the total costs of residency programs.

TABLE 3.4   HMO Enrollment (millions)

MEMBERSHIP	1990	1992	1995	2000
Individual HMO	28	44	56	100
Medicare HMO	1	3	7	18
Medicaid HMO	—	—	5	20

Source: Coile, R.C. (1995). Assessing healthcare market trends and capital needs, 1996–2000. *Healthcare Financial Management, August,* 60–62.

Given the federal government's commitment to reducing Medicare spending and the need to add incentives for primary care, payments to hospitals for graduate medical education (GME) are a prime target for savings. Current proposals under consideration take the form of limiting reimbursement for specialists, requiring a set percentage of residency positions to be in family practice or internal medicine, and requiring that a defined percent of training take place in outpatient or community settings.

MARKET DEMAND

The forces briefly discussed in the preceding section—recognition of the oversupply of physicians and overuse of specialists, mismatch between the characteristics of the modern acute care system and the needs and characteristics of the current patient population, and the mandate to reduce costs—have combined to create a demand for change in the fundamental way in which acute care is provided. However, while there is agreement about the need for change, there is little consensus about the degree of redesign required, with some arguing that minor adjustments to the work force is all that is required, while others suggest that we should be envisioning a more radical change.

The clearest description and the best understood reason for the creation of the ACNP role is as a response to a market demand for an expanded or altered work force. This demand is very real and probably accounts for the rapidity of developments in this area. It is essentially a call for a new member of the work force who can meet several needs—replacement or substitute for house staff, shepherd, and quality improvement manager.

Altered Work Force

This very apparent and forceful demand for ACNPs stems from the changes occurring and projected for the next decade in the physician work force. The trends in health care that have affected the demand for physician services include the national consensus that total supply of physicians is excessive, that the distribution of the types of physicians is ineffective for accessible, cost-effective care, and that the number of specialists needs to decrease and the number of generalists needs to increase (Cooper, 1994; Weiner, 1993; Shine, 1995). However, despite the agreement in principle that there is an excess number of physicians, graduate medical trainees increased by more than 15% from 1988–1993 (Epstein, 1995). Thus, the need to downsize residency programs to reduce the oversupply of physicians and change the focus of training from specialists to generalists continues to be acute and the inevitable changes will be rather dramatic. The decrease in Medicare funding, described earlier, will facilitate movement toward downsizing internal medicine programs (Asch & Ende, 1992), as will the greater emphasis on training in primary care proposed by the Council on Graduate Medical Education and the Association of American Medical Colleges (Stoddard, Kindig, & Libby, 1994).

The decrease in reimbursement for medical education by decreased Medicare funding will profoundly affect not only the ability to support graduate medical education, but also the viability of teaching hospitals which rely on house staff in training to care for patients (Inglehart, 1994). The expense of house staff training and research in teaching hospitals increases the costs of care 20% over those of nonteaching hospitals. Thus, teaching hospitals in particular need to lower costs to stay competitive and to use alternative, less expensive, providers of direct care at the bedside. Changes in the composition, number and availability of the physician work force will leave vacancies in patient care managers in the hospital.

In addition to concern about the numbers of direct care providers, there is growing recognition that the current model of using physicians-in-training as the major provider of care in tertiary settings is fundamentally flawed. The efficiency of the traditional role of medical residents and their ability to meet both the service needs of the hospital and their own educational needs has obvious implications for cost and quality of care. Medical residents have the dual objective of providing patient care and meeting learning needs; this has several implications. First, significant amounts of the resident's time each day must be spent in educational activities rather than patient care. Second, there is an incentive for the resident to practice new skills, gain experience with procedures, and to overuse diagnostic testing. Third, like any novice, the resident's overall efficiency is likely to be quite low until he or she has gained some experience in the area. All of these sources of inefficiency would be eliminated if residents were allowed to concentrate on their learning needs, while another type of expert clinician was utilized to provide the direct care or service function. This is a key element of the rationale for using ACNPs in place of interns and residents.

The need for a skilled practitioner is also evident in hospitals that do not have residency programs. In these nonteaching hospitals, physicians must rely on staff nurses and rotational or "house" physicians to facilitate patients' plans of care in their absence. Staff nurses do not have the advanced education required to manage patient care and house physicians focus on meeting only the immediate patient care needs rather than facilitating diagnosis, discharge planning, or referrals. In both teaching and nonteaching hospitals, physicians and nurses have become accustomed to developing separate plans of care with separate medical and nursing interventions. The lack of integration of medical and nursing interventions has the potential for leaving gaps in patient care that are particularly troublesome in our current environment of increased patient acuity and complexity. Both models of care in the teaching and nonteaching hospital, with traditional physician-nurse relationships, represent inefficient ways to care for acutely ill patients that have great potential for fragmented, costly care.

Thus, there is an eminent demand for a care provider who can meet the needs of the current and changing health care system in the inpatient setting. Historically nurses have expanded their scope of practice to respond to patient needs for increased access to primary health care. To address advanced practice issues for patients with specialized needs in the past, the primary care NP and the CNS roles were developed. Nurses are now being called upon again to meet patient needs in a costly system with inadequate numbers of care providers.

The breadth of NP preparation which builds on a foundation of nursing experience and encompasses advanced assessment, differential diagnostic skills and treatment strategies makes the ACNP the logical choice. The role and scope of practice of ACNP fulfills the needs for a substitute/replacement for house staff physicians and an expert clinician to address system inefficiencies. Since ACNPs are no longer students and do not have the need to be exposed to a wide variety of patients and procedures as part of their formal educational program, they actually become more expert at caring for specific patient populations and at some of the technological aspects related to specific patient populations (Keane & Richmond, 1993; Clochesy, Daly, Idemoto, Steel, & Fitzpatrick, 1994). ACNPs quickly become skilled in their field and competent to deliver expert care rather than moving on to new training ground. The American College of Physicians supports the nurse practitioner (NP) role as substitute for house staff in the inpatient setting (American College of Physicians, 1994) and the American Nurses Association supports this advanced role through the development of the Standards and Scope of Practice for the Acute Care Nurse Practitioner and, most recently, a national certification examination (American Association of Critical Care Nurses & American Nurses Association, 1995).

Nurse practitioners have practiced in inpatient settings for many years but most have typically practiced within the pediatric or speciality services such as trauma surgery (Silver, Murphy, & Gitterman, 1984; Spisso, O'Callaghan, McKennan, & Holcroft, 1990; Dale, 1991). Much of the literature on inpatient NPs focuses on a model which conceives of the role only as a substitute or replacement for medical residents in teaching hospitals (Honigfeld, Perloff, & Barzansky, 1990; Knickman, Lipkin, Finkler, Thompson, & Kiel, 1992; Nemes, Barnaby, & Shamberger, 1992; Silver & McAtee, 1984, 1988). One study, which evaluated the use of NPs as replacement for house staff in a teaching childrens' hospital, confirmed the ability of the NP to provide safe, efficient care in an acute care environment (Nemes, Barnaby, & Shamberger, 1992). Institution of the NP role decreased residents' workloads, improved communication between surgeons and their patients, and increased time for surgical resident education and learning. Another study conducted on a trauma service in a teaching hospital found that with implementation of the NP role costs decreased, quality of care improved and the health care team worked more efficiently and communicated more effectively (Spisso, O'Callaghan, McKennan, & Holcroft, 1990). Lastly, substitution of NPs and PAs was surveyed in 389 hospitals that were members of the Council of Teaching Hospitals in a study by the Robert Wood Johnson Foundation. The results revealed that (1) although more facilities used PAs, their number and that of the NPs was about equal and (2) that NPs substituted on average for third-year residents while PAs substituted for second-year residents (Riportella-Muller, Libby, & Kindig, 1994).

The question of who should substitute for physicians—NPs or PAs—is one that is frequently debated in discussions about how to manage the workload in the face of decreasing numbers of interns and residents in acute care. Responding to this question requires careful, objective consideration of the similarities and differences between NPs and PAs.

There are notable similarities in the histories of the NP and PA roles. Both originated in the 1960s, spurred by the need to expand availability of affordable primary care services and increased access to health care for the medically underserved. The first educational programs for both roles were certificate programs combining intensive didactic material in the basic sciences with a full-time, precepted clinical experience. Over the next decade, guidelines and criteria for educational programs were developed and today most PA and NP programs are associated with medical centers and universities.

Currently, 62.5% of PA programs award a baccalaureate degree and 16% award a master's degree upon completion (Oliver, 1993). The rest award either an associate's degree or a certificate of completion. All graduates must sit for a national certifying examination following graduation from an AMA-approved program. Curricula typically involve a series of courses in basic and behavioral sciences and professional issues, didactic clinical courses, and clinical clerkships or rotations. The most common baccalaureate program design includes two years of preclinical academic course work, followed by two years of clinical experience (Fowkes, 1993).

It is difficult to compare PA and NP programs because of the wide variation among them. There are some clear differences, however, related to the ways in which these programs have developed and the status of most NP programs as postgraduate or master's degree programs. Physician assistant programs were originally, and to a great extent still are, strongly oriented toward primary care, whereas basic nursing programs have been much broader, aimed at preparing the beginning practitioner for all possible sites of practice. The average NP has gained several years of experience working in a staff nurse role before returning to school for graduate education as an NP. Thus, the typical NP is likely to have a broader base of preparation, particularly in the behavioral sciences, and considerable patient care experience before assuming the role of practitioner.

Perhaps more important, the role of the PA has always been conceptualized as existing in a close, dependent relationship with physicians, improving access to care for patients by serving as physician extenders. The American Medical Association retains control of PA education through its accreditation program. Nursing, particularly in the past few decades, has consciously and aggressively worked toward recognition of its status as an independent profession based upon a unique body of knowledge. In general, nurses are educated to work in close collaboration with physicians and other health care workers but do not see their practice as having any necessary dependence on the practice of other professionals. In contrast to characteristics of PAs, the existence of a separate professional nursing organization, control of the accreditation process by an independent nursing organization (National League for Nursing), and licensing by state boards of nursing reflects this philosophy.

The issue of similarities and differences between NPs and PAs must be understood in light of the functions of each. If we conceive of the ACNP as merely a substitute for the physician, it is unlikely that we will find significant differences in the competence and performance of NPs and PAs. Experience in primary care has shown that both types of clinicians perform equally well and that both can be an effective substitute for about 70–80% of tasks or patient encounters (Spitzer, et al., 1974; Cawley, 1993; Office of Technology Assessment, 1987; Safriet, 1992). It is reasonable to assume that these same figures would apply to the substitution of NPs and PAs in acute care. However, this approach to assessing these roles is inadequate to the objectives of improving the functioning of the acute care system and the care delivered to patients in these systems. It is in the roles of shepherd and quality improvement facilitator that the differences between NPs and PAs are most apparent.

Shepherd Role

Though we have an acute care system that offers the newest and most sophisticated technology, there is growing dissatisfaction by consumers and health care providers with the need to navigate complex and disjointed services. Care is often fragmented for patients who are repeatedly hospitalized for exacerbations of chronic health problems even though they may be familiar with the system. For patients with new health problems who are unfamiliar with the system, exposure to repeated examinations and questioning by novices and their supervisors, coping with the many specialists, facing the variety of decisions that must be made regarding treatment choices and the rapidity with which discharge arrangements must be made is often overwhelming. The frequent absence of a primary care provider or someone to coordinate plans among specialists and ancillary medical services leaves patients and their families at great risk of both iatrogenic harms and ineffective treatment regimens.

Addressing these needs requires a professional who is academically prepared to make thorough assessments and to understand the complex disease processes and sophisticated treatments used as well as patient responses to their illnesses. In addition, a clinician who is knowledgeable about the resources available and how to make them accessible is needed. These are the skills which the ACNP brings to the situation of acute care. Acute care nurse practitioners are qualified to manage the medical and nursing care of patients at the bedside, carry out a substitutive physician role, and to act as "shepherd" or guide through the foreign maze of the hospital system.

This shepherd role is delineated within the Standards of Clinical Practice for the ACNP (AACN & ANA, 1995). The expectations outlined in the Standards encompass the facilitation of organizational resources in caring for the patient. This aspect of the NP role helps patients and families understand the complicated system of consultants and/or specialists, interdisciplinary services such as occupational therapy, physical therapy, respiratory therapy, dietary services and social services as well as facilitate the transition from the outpatient setting to the inpatient setting and back. In doing so, the ACNP ensures both efficiency of care and effectiveness of services.

The preparation and background of NPs makes them ideally prepared to assume this shepherd role. While physicians have traditionally focused on the medical model of disease and cure, nurses have focused on models of health and care. Medicine has made wonderful strides in improving quality patient care through new and better medical treatments, but this narrow focus is simply not sufficient to address the current deficits in our acute care system. Nurses have long been committed to improving quality patient care by responding to human responses to illness, regardless of whether these responses consist of physiologic symptoms, subjective complaints, or social welfare needs.

In the acute care setting, patients are more likely to have acute physiologic problems which demand astute assessment and immediate medical intervention. Thus the initial plan is typically focused on the patient's medical problem. Acute care nurse practitioners are not only experienced in assessing and evaluating physiological parameters but also experienced in assessing psychosocial, cultural and religious factors which may contribute to the illness or health problems. This leads to a plan of care focused on a combination of what have traditionally been understood as nursing and medical problems. Knowledge of the infinite variety of contributing factors allows the NP to help patients identify interventions related to their immediate health problem and health maintenance activities that are compatible and realistic in terms of lifestyle and financial status and effective in preventing new health problems. The focus on care not cure is the commitment of all professional nurses.

An example may illustrate how the ACNP can effectively shepherd an acutely ill patient through the hospital system. One of the most common diagnoses seen in acute care is myocardial infarction (MI). When caring for the MI patient, the ACNP will most likely initiate a care path. Care paths and protocols have become increasingly essential in capitated health systems. While all members of the care team can utilize the care path in guiding interventions, effective use requires careful assessment of the need for exceptions and monitoring variances. Staff nurses may need assistance in detecting subtle changes or identifying needed alterations in a timely manner, while residents who rotate through specialty areas and physicians who admit patients to several different hospitals may be unfamiliar with the protocol itself. The NP who works in the cardiac care unit will have expert knowledge of the needs of MI patients, the diagnostic tests that need to be ordered on schedule to confirm or rule out the diagnosis, and the usual approach to symptom management. Knowledge of the established time-line for progression to a telemetry unit or general division will assist in moving the patient through the system on schedule. Further, the ACNP's understanding of the pathophysiology and etiology of the disease will enable him or her to assess the patient's lifestyle and identify needs for patient and family teaching.

This example illustrates how APN's can facilitate continuity of care and how familiarity with system issues can facilitate efficient diagnosis, treatment and referrals for follow-up care. In assuming these responsibilities, the ACNP does not obviate the patient's need for expert medical care, but rather supplements the physician's and staff nurse's care and makes the process of care more effective. Acute care nurse practitioners are able to bridge the gap between nursing and medicine and thus incorporate cure and care by fusing previously separate and uncoordinated nursing and medical plans. Giacalone, Mullaney, DeJoseph, and Cosma's (1995) recent description of a program using a blended CNS-NP role in a cardiac access unit is an excellent example of putting this role to work in improving coordination of care.

Quality Improvement Manager

The last way in which ACNPs can complement rather than merely substitute for physicians is in quality-monitoring activities. The components of total quality management, total quality improvement and quality assurance are well known to nurses. Much of the focus of these "quality improvement" activities in the past has been driven by regulatory bodies and by the objective of cost containment. However, the focus of these narrow quality assurance programs has expanded recently with better understanding of the need to integrate quality improvement techniques both as part of routine operations and particularly with any redesign program.

As nurses, ACNPs are expert at examining policy and practice issues that affect outcomes and determine quality of care. Again, the APN's background in group leadership, program administration, and familiarity with interdepartmental and interdisciplinary efforts enable him or her to contribute to the design and implementation of continuous quality improvement programs. Nurses, probably more than any other hospital staff member, are quite knowledgeable about the interworkings of the many departments involved in patient care and areas or processes in need of streamlining.

Some may argue that these last two functions (shepherd and quality improvement facilitator) are aspects of case management. They are indeed part of effective case management. They are separated here in order to more precisely describe the ways in which the ACNP role entails more than substitution for reduced numbers of residents. It also helps to explain why it is essential that educational programs for ACNPs include more than just clinical preparation. If the ACNP is going to be prepared to function effectively in the redesigned acute care system of the future, he or she must continue to be prepared as a systems expert.

UNRESOLVED ISSUES

Barriers to Practice

Although there is no question that the ACNP role can meet the demand for a new type of acute care provider, there continue to be significant barriers to NPs in the current system. The experience of primary care NPs can be instructive in both understanding and responding to these barriers. In a recent study, Hupcey (1993) surveyed NPs regarding those factors in the workplace that either hindered or supported practice in a variety of settings, including hospitals. She found that, while acceptance by MDs was mentioned most frequently as a helping factor, followed by support from co-workers, the factor that most often hindered practice was lack of administrative support. This underscores the importance of taking steps to prepare the environments where our students will work as part of ensuring their success following graduation.

Among the negative factors most commonly faced by NPs are lack of understanding of the role and concern about encroaching on others' practice. These are perceived as lack of support from administrators and colleagues, both medical and nursing. A great deal of education and information sharing must take place in the practice arena in order to prepare the environment for the arrival of ACNPs.

A strategy that can be quite effective is to approach the establishment of this role as a marketing project. The key, of course, to any marketing project is to identify those aspects of the "product" that are needed or desired by the consumer and to then package and advertise the product in these terms. So, when we talk with administrators we want to emphasize how these practitioners can lead to cost savings. This is not obvious because the direct cost of ACNPs always exceeds that of house staff. However, house staff, while inexpensive in terms of salary, are quite expensive in terms of inefficiencies. There are some data in the literature that have documented the expense associated with utilization of house staff as managers of care. Most of these studies have taken place in critical care units (Daly, Rudy, Thompson, & Happ, 1991; Roberts, Ostryznink, & McEwen, 1991; Zimmerman et al, 1993), but combining these findings with Barbara Safriet's (1992) excellent review of data related to cost savings associated with advanced practice nursing and Nichols' (1992) model of the cost of underutilizing APNs can make a convincing case.

In talking with physicians and nurses, however, emphasizing the cost savings to the system is unlikely to be persuasive. When we talk with our physician colleagues, we must emphasize how adding NPs to the inpatient team will reduce demands on house staff and perhaps solve the problem of how to accomplish as much with fewer house officers. With nursing colleagues, it can be effective to talk about how working with clinicians who are also nurses and share the same perspective and priorities will make the job of the staff nurse easier and will enable them to more readily meet their patient's needs.

Although these approaches can be effective with most professionals, unfortunately there is considerable misunderstanding and opposition to the continued evolution of all advanced nursing practice roles, including that of the ACNP. Since the first pediatric NP programs in the 1970s, debate has continued regarding the appropriateness and safety of primary care NPs. Fottler, Gibson, and Pinchoff (1978) documented the prevalence of opposition to NPs among 944 physicians. The four major reasons for physician unwillingness to employ an NP were perceived lack of applicability of the role to their specialty (35.3% of respondents), satisfaction with traditional roles and relationships (26.6%), concern about legal liability (17.9%), and perceived inability of the NP to perform in an expanded role

(17.9%). In discussing physician opposition, the authors noted that "the medical community is hospitable to innovations which conform to previously upheld values, but inhospitable to those which require emancipation from these values (p. 304)." Almost 20 years later, little has changed. The 1995 *Guidelines for Physicians/Nurse Practitioners Integrated Practice* (AMA, 1995) include the following points: "(1) The *physician* is responsible for managing the health care of patients . . . (4) The extent of involvement by the nurse practitioner in initial assessment, and implementation of treatment will depend on the complexity and acuity of the patients' condition *as determined by the physician* (italics added)."

Almost two decades later, this same resistance to change is still apparent in segments of both the nursing and medical professions. Despite the publication of a great number of studies documenting the effectiveness of NPs, there continues to be strong opposition from organized medicine, reflected in what Inglis and Kjervik term "conflicting and restrictive provisions governing [advanced practice nurses'] scope of practice and prescriptive authority, as well as the parsimonious and fragmented state and federal standards for reimbursement" (Inglis & Kjervik, 1993). The strength of the personal feelings engendered by the NP movement are evident in the many published professional editorials and letters on this subject (Can APNs be independent gatekeepers, 1993; DeAngelis, 1994; Fightlin, 1994; Kassirer, 1994; LePage, 1994; Anonymous, 1994) as well as discussions in the lay press (Nurses' lib, 1993; Petty, 1993; Weisskopf, 1993; Wolf, 1993). Thus, it is essential that the resistance to the needed growth and utilization of the ACNP role not be underestimated. Like all major social changes, establishment of this role and support of the newest practitioners will require very careful and persistent work by the profession as a whole as well as by individual educators and administrators.

Regulation

Regulation is the last issue that is crucial to implementing the vision of how the role of the ACNP can contribute to patient care. As with specific features of the work environment, the status of regulation has a major impact on the role of the ACNP and thus has to be a consideration in how the ACNP role fits within the current system.

There are currently a number of ways in which we do and do not regulate advanced practice (Pearson, 1993). Sixteen states require a separate, additional license as authorization for some forms of advanced practice. Twenty-two states govern practice through regulations establishing a certification procedure, and 19 states issue some kind of letter or other written authorization (National Council of State Boards of Nursing, 1993). Some states use a combination of methods. And unfortunately, we still have a few states, such as Ohio and Illinois, where advanced practice is not recognized.

Like much of nursing, this diversity is somewhat problematic to both the practitioner and consumer. However, we have failed to reach any consensus in the profession concerning which method of regulation is most appropriate. One of the most divisive questions concerns the requirement for a second or additional advanced practice license. The arguments in favor requiring APNs to obtain an additional license include:

- licensure is the clearest form of regulation; its meaning is evident to all
- licensure is considered the most restrictive form of authorization and thus it provides the strongest form of protection of the consumer from incompetent practitioners; licensure generally carries regulations regarding revocation, a process not usually included in certification systems
- licensing laws usually provide title protection
- the regulations establishing licensing usually place the authority for granting licensure within the State Board of Nursing, where the authority rightly belongs.

Arguments against second licensure include:

- the restrictiveness does not protect the consumer any better than do certification rules and it may place undue burdens upon the professional trying to qualify
- State boards are political bodies, not professional; membership often includes non-nurses
- scope of practice should be defined by the professional body— the ANA

- licensure is not universally the sole domain of the State Boards of Nursing; in many states this authority is shared by Boards of Medicine.

There is little correlation between the stringency of regulations and licensure. Certification rules are necessarily more lax. In addition to the variation in overall approach, there is also quite a bit of variation in the specific rules. Some states maintain a list of approved schools and applicants must either graduate from an approved program or petition to have their specific program approved before certification will be granted. Other states simply require graduation from an advanced practice program (which does not, in every case, have to be at the graduate level) and passing a certification exam.

While the debate about regulation continues, the implications for educators include the need to be knowledgeable not just about the requirements in their own states, but also in surrounding states. For example, most states have specific requirements for a specific number of hours of pharmacology preparation as part of eligibility for prescriptive authority. Consequently, inclusion of 45 hours of pharmacology content in the ACNP curriculum is recommended. Educators must remain knowledgeable about trends in regulation such as this so that the current variation in state requirements does not become an additional barrier to practice.

SUMMARY

This chapter has discussed some of the more significant characteristics of the current health care system that have contributed to the demand for ACNP. These characteristics include trends in the profession of medicine, needs of the current patient population, and mandates to reduce cost. The most apparent and strongest market demand is for a replacement of the decreasing numbers of interns and residents who will be available in the future for patient care in acute care hospitals. However, we can also rely on ACNPs to shepherd patients through the maze of tertiary-care facilities and to participate in modifying the health care system to make lasting improvements.

REFERENCES

Aiken, L. (1995). Medicare funding of nursing education. *Journal of the American Medical Association, 273*, 1528–1532.

American Association of Colleges of Nursing. (1993). *Nursing education's agenda for the 21st century*. Washington, DC: AACN.

American Association of Critical Care Nurses & American Nurses Association. (1995). *Scope of practice for the acute care nurse practitioner and the standards of clinical practice for the acute care nurse practitioner*. Washington, DC: American Nurses Association.

American College of Physicians. (1994). Physician assistants and nurse practitioners. *Annals of Internal Medicine, 121*, 714–716.

American Medical Association. (1995). *Guidelines for Physicians'/Nurse Practitioners' integrated practice*. CMS Report 15 (I-94), Chicago: American Medical Association.

American Nurses Association. (1995). *Managed care curriculum*. Washington, DC: Author.

Anonymous. (1994, May). Letter to the editor. *American Nurse*, p. 3.

Asch, D. A., & Ende, J. (1992). The downsizing of internal medicine residency. *Annals of Internal Medicine, 117*(10), 839–844.

Babbott, D., Levey, G. S., Weaver, S. O., & Killian, C. D. (1991). Medical students attitudes about internal medicine: A study of the U.S. medical school seniors in 1988. *Annals of Internal Medicine, 114*, 16–22.

Bluestone, N. (1993). The bottom line. *Journal of the American Medical Association, 269*, 2580.

Brooten, D. (1993). Assisting with transitions from hospital to home. In S. G. Funk, E. M. Tornquist, M. T. Champagne, & R. A. Wiese, Eds., *Key aspects of caring for the chronically ill*. New York: Springer Publishing Co., 30–37.

Can APNs be independent gatekeepers? (1993, June 5). *Hospitals and Health Networks*, p. 8.

Cawley, J. F. (1993). Physician assistants in the health care workforce. In D. K. Clawson & M. Osterweis, Eds., *Roles of physician assistants and nurse practitioners in primary care*. Washington, DC: Association of Academic Health Centers, 21–38.

Clochesy, J. M., Daly, B. J., Idemoto, B. K., Steel, J., & Fitzpatrick, J. J. (1994). Preparing Advanced Practice Nurses for acute care. *American Journal of Critical Care, 3*(4), 255–258.

Coile, R. C. (1995). Assessing healthcare market trends and capital needs, 1996–2000. *Healthcare Financial Management, August,* 60–62.

Commission on Professional and Hospital Activities. (1986). *Lengths of stay: Geriatric length of stay by diagnosis and operation, U.S., 1985.* Ann Arbor, MI: Author.

Committee on Ways and Means, U.S. House of Representatives. (1991). *Health care resource book.* Washington, DC: U.S. Government Printing Office.

Cooper, R. A. (1994). Seeking a balanced physician workforce for the 21st century. *Journal of the American Medical Association, 272*(9), 680–687.

Dale, J. C. (1991). New role for PNPs in an inpatient setting. *J Ped Health Care, 5*(6), 336.

Daly, B. J., Rudy, E. B., Thompson, K. S., & Happ, M. B. (1991). Development of a special care unit for chronically critically ill patients. *Heart and Lung, 20,* 45–51.

DeAngelis, C. D. (1994). Nurse practitioner redux. *Journal of the American Medical Association, 271,* 868–871.

DeBois, A., & Kjervik, D. K. (1993). Empowerment of advanced practice nurses: Regulation reform needed to increase access to care. *Journal of Law, Medicine, Ethics, 21*(2), 193–205.

Epstein, A. M. (1995). U.S. teaching hospitals in the evolving health care spectrum. *Journal of the American Medical Association, 273*(15), 1203–1207.

Fightlin, M. L. (1994). Letter to the editor. *Journal of the American Medical Association, 272,* 592.

Fottler, M. D., Gibson, G., & Pinchoff, D. M. (1978). Physician attitudes towards the nurse practitioner. *Journal of Health and Social Behavior, 19,* 303–311.

Fowkes, V. (1993). Meeting the needs of the underserved: The roles of physician assistants and nurse practitioners. In D. K. Clawson & M. Osterweis, Eds., *Roles of physician assistants and nurse practitioners in primary care.* Washington, DC: Association of Academic Health Centers, 69–83.

Giacalone, M. B., Mullaney, D., DeJoseph, D. A., & Cosma, M. (1995). Development of a nurse-managed unit and the advanced practitioner role. *Critical Care Clinics of North America, 7*(1), 35–41.

Goksel, D., Harrison, C. J., Morrison, R. E., & Miller, S. T. (1993). Description of a nurse practitioner inpatient service in a public teaching hospital. *Journal of General Internal Medicine, 8,* 29–30.

Havre, D. C. (1993). Intimacy in medicine. *Journal of the Florida Medical Association*, *80*, 281–282.

Health United States, 1992. (1993). Hyattsville, MD: Department of Health and Human Services, National Center for Health Statistics. DHHS Pub. No. (PHS) 93-1232.

Honigfeld, L., Perloff, J., & Barzansky, B. (1990). Replacing the work of pediatric residents: Strategies and issues. *Pediatrics*, *85*(6), 969–976.

Hupcey, J. E. (1993). Factors and work settings that may influence nurse practitioner practice. *Nursing Outlook*, *41*, 181–5.

Inglehart, J. K. (1994). Health policy report: Rapid changes for academic medical centers. *New England Journal of Medicine*, *331*(20), 1391–1395.

Ingtis, A. D., & Kjervik, D. K. (1993). Empowerment of advanced practice nurses: Regulation reform needed to increase access to care. *Journal of Law, Medicine, & Ethics, 21*, 193–205.

Johnson, S. J. (1994). GME financing: a well-kept secret. *Nursing Management*, *25*(4), 43–46.

Kassirer, J. K. (1994). Waht role for nurse practitioners in primary care? *New England Journal of Medicine*, *330*, 204–205.

Keane, A., & Richmond, T. (1993). Tertiary nurse practitioners. *Image*, *25*(4), 281–284.

Knickman, J. R., Lipkin, M., Finkler, S. A., Thompson, W. G., & Kiel, J. (1992). The potential for using non-physicians to compensate for the reduced availability of residents. *Academic Medicine*, *67*(7), 429–438.

Koepper, L. L., Mess, M. A., & Troff, K. J. (1995). Planning for managed care. *Healthcare Financial Management, November*, 44–47.

Lepage, M. (1994). Letter to the editor. *Journal of the American Medical Association*, *272*, 592.

Marwick, C. (1994). Preservation of physician-patient relationship seen as integral to health care system reform. *Journal of the American Medical Association, 271*, 892–893.

National Council of State Boards of Nursing. (1993). *Fact Sheet.* Chicago: National Council of State Boards of Nursing, Inc.

Nemes, J., Barnaby, K., & Shamberger, R. (1992). Experience with a nurse practitioner program in the surgical department of a children's hospital. *Journal of Pediatric Surgery*, *27*(8), 1038–1042.

Nichols, L. M. (1992). Estimating costs of underutilizing advanced practice nurses. *Nursing Economics*, *10*(5), 343–351.

Nurses' lib. (1993, August 13). *Wall Street Journal*, p. B4.

Office of Technology Assessment. (1986). *Nurse practitioner, physician assistant and certified nurse midwives: A policy analysis.* Health technology case study #37. Washington, DC: U.S. Government Printing Office.

Office of Technology Assessment, United States Congress. (1987). *Life-sustaining technologies and the elderly*. Washington, DC: U.S. Government Printing office, OTA-BA-306.

Oliver, D. (1993). Physician assistant education: a review of program characteristics by sponsoring institution. In D. K. Clawson & M. Osterweis, Eds., *Roles of physician assistants and nurse practitioners in primary care*. Washington, DC: Association of Academic Health Centers, 85–110.

Pearson, L. J. (1993). 1992–93 update: How each state stands on legislative issues affecting advanced nursing practice. *Nurse Practitioner, 18*(1), 23–38.

Petersdorf, R. G. (1993). Primary care—medical students' unpopular choice. *American Journal of Public Health, 83*, 328–330.

Petty, A. (1993, September 2). Nurse practitioners fight job restrictions. *Wall Street Journal*, pp. B1, B3.

Prospective Payment Assessment Commission. (June 1994). *Medicare and the American health system report to congress*. Washington, DC: Author.

Riportella-Muller, R., Libby, D., & Kindig, D. (January, 1994). The national experience with the substitution of physician assistants and nurse practitioners for medical residents in Council of Teaching Hospitals member hospitals. Unpublished report to the Robert Wood Johnson Foundation.

Roberts, D., Ostryznink, T., & McEwen, T. (1991). Effect of a resource management system on ICU laboratory utilization. *American Review of Respiratory Disease, 143* (Inter. Conf. Supp., Abstracts): A 469, 143.

Safriet, B. J. (1992). Health care dollars and regulatory sense: the role of advanced practice nursing. *Yale Journal on Regulation, 9*, 417–487.

Schwartz, M. D., Linzer, M., Babbott, D., Divine, G. W., Broadhead, E., & the Society of General Internal Medicine Interest Group on Career Choice in Internal Medicine. (1991). Medical student interest in internal medicine. *Annals of Internal Medicine, 114*(1), 6–15.

Shine, K. I. (1995). Freeze the number of Medicare subsidized graduate medical education positions. *Journal of the American Medical Association, 273*(13), 1057–58.

Silver, H. K., & McAtee, P. (1984). The use of nonphysician "associate residents" in overcrowded speciality-training program. *New England Journal of Medicine, 311*, 326–328.

Silver, H. K., & McAtee, P. (1988). Should nurse substitute for house staff? *American Journal of Nursing, 88*, 1671–1673.

Silver, H. K., Murphy, M. A., Gitterman, B. A. (1984). The hospital nurse practitioner in pediatrics. *American Journal of Diseases of Children*, *138*, 237–239.

Spisso, J., O'Callaghan, C, McKennan, M., & Holcroft, J. W. (1990). Improved quality of care and the reduction of housestaff workload using trauma nurse practitioners. *Journal of Trauma*, *30*(6), 660–665.

Spitzer, W. O., Sackett, D. L., Sibley, J. C., Roberts, R. S., Gent, M., Kergin, D. J., Hackett, B. C., & Olynich, A. (1974). The Burlington randomized trial of nurse practitioners. *New England Journal of Medicine*, *290*(5), 251–256.

Stoddard, J. J., Kindig, D. A., & Libby, D. (1994). Graduate medical education reform: Service provision transition costs. *Journal of the American Medical Association*, *272*(1), 53–58.

United States Department of Commerce, Bureau of the Census. (1983). *America in transition: An aging society*. Washington, DC: U.S. Government Printing Office, Series P-23, No. 128.

Weiner, J. P. (1993). The demand for physician services in a changing health care system: A synthesis. *Medical Care Review*, *50*(4), 411–449.

Weisskopf, M. (1993, May 16). In health debate, nurses exerting powers of numbers and purses. *Washington Post*, pp. A1, A16.

Wennberg, J. E., Goodman, D. C., Nease, R. F., & Keller, R. B. (1993). Finding equilibrium in U.S. physician supply. *Health Affairs, Summer 1993*, 91–103.

Wolf, C. (1993, September 20). Expanding duties for nurses prompts debate. *Crain's Cleveland Business*, pp. 22–23.

Zimmerman, J. E., Shortell, S. M., Knaus, W. A., Rousseau, D. M., Wagner, D. P., Gillies, R. R., Draper, E. A., & Devers, K. (1993). Value and cost of teaching hospitals: A prospective, multicenter, inception cohort study. *Critical Care Medicine*, *21*(10), 1432–1442.

Chapter **4**

EDUCATIONAL STANDARDS FOR ACNPs

John M. Clochesy, PhD, RN, FCCM, FAAN
Barbara J. Daly, PhD, RN, FAAN

Educational standards for ACNPs are dynamic and continually evolving, as is the ACNP role itself. Initially educational programs to prepare ACNPs resulted from the urgent demand for APNs prepared to function in the acute care setting. These early programs drew from the expertise of individual schools in preparing either acute care clinical nurse specialists or primary care NPs. With the rapid increase in interest in these programs came an appreciation of the need to carefully consider standards for educating the ACNP.

In response to this need, a series of consensus conferences were held to identify if there was general agreement about what a curriculum should include to prepare APNs for acute care (Standards for Educational Programs, 1994). The first conference, held in Boston in the spring of 1993, drew 47 participants, representing 11 academic institutions, 9 clinical agencies, and 5 professional nursing organizations. The second conference, held in Cleveland in 1994, grew to 87 participants, representing 30 institutions and organizations. These consensus conferences were hosted by participants on a voluntary basis. Beginning with the 4th Annual Consensus Conference, a national planning committee was formed to ensure the broadest possible representation in the development of these important meetings.

Although existing consensus regarding education for the ACNP role has been heavily influenced by the discussions at these national meetings, program development has been importantly directed by the larger context of the history of NP and clinical nurse specialist education, funding patterns for advanced practice education, and the views and activities of professional nursing organizations. This chapter therefore will briefly review these influences before discussing the current level of agreement about ACNP programs.

NURSE PRACTITIONER AND CLINICAL NURSE SPECIALIST EDUCATION

As discussed by Steel in chapter 2, education of NPs had moved from the early pattern of continuing education programs to university-based master's degree programs by the 1990s. This movement has been formally sanctioned by the requirement of the largest certifying body, the American Nurses Credentialing Center, that as of 1997 candidates for certification will have to be prepared in either a master's degree NP program or a postgraduate program granting graduate academic credit (American Nurses Credentialing Center, 1995a).

Trends in NP education have been marked by the publication of two important documents. In 1972, the *Federal Guidelines for Preparation of Nurse Practitioners* was published, representing early standards regarding content of NP programs. These guidelines were viewed as necessary because of the rapid proliferation of NP programs offered by a variety of providers, including schools of nursing, hospitals, and commercial continuing education organizations (Secretary's Committee, 1972). With this as a base, consensus developed regarding core content of NP programs. Mezey (1993, p. 49) summarizes the categories of this core as follows:

1. The philosophy and concepts underlying NP practice
2. The NP's role within the health care system
3. The scientific base for NP functioning
4. Components of role implementation
5. Common management concerns of NPs.

More recently, the National Organization of Nurse practitioner Faculties (NONPF) published its *Advanced Nursing Practice: Nurse Practitioner Curriculum Guidelines* (Zimmer et al., 1990). These guidelines provide the organization's recommendations regarding curriculum content, requirements for clinical practicums, faculty qualifications, and desired competencies for graduates of all types of NP programs, although they were written primarily with primary care providers in mind.

Recommendations from NONPF that have been most important in influencing the direction of ACNP curricula are the identification of the domains of practice and the standards for clinical experiences of students. *The Guidelines* delineate five domains of practice for nurse practitioners:

- management of client health/illness status
- monitoring and ensuring the quality of health care practice
- organizational and role competencies
- the healing role of the nurse
- the teaching-coaching function of the nurse.

In addition to *The Guidelines*, NONPF has also developed standards for "model programs." These standards include a requirement for a minimum of 600 hours of clinical practice for students. Although specifications in NONPF's *Guidelines* and *Model Program* are not formally part of certification processes or graduate program evaluations, they do set an important reference standard for faculty designing and teaching in ACNP programs (Boodley, 1995b).

Existing curricula of clinical nurse specialist (CNS) programs have had a direct impact on ACNP curricula in two ways. First, as discussed in more detail in the first two chapters of this book, opinion regarding the appropriateness of merging the roles of ACNP and CNS into one advanced practice role versus the need to maintain separate roles and competencies continues to be divided. Schools that have adopted the philosophy that the health care system will not support distinct roles in the future have modified existing CNS curricula, usually by adding more content supporting the direct care function of the APN, such as initiating a separate course in pharmacology and adding more clinical hours. Content supporting the indirect functions, such as teaching and consultation, has sometimes been reduced to maintain total program credits at the same level.

Even schools that have not made an explicit decision to merge role preparation have usually designed their first ACNP curricula from core content believed to be common to all advanced practice roles. Thus their CNS and ACNP programs differ only in the clinical courses.

Beliefs of faculty regarding the issue of role fusion will continue to be a central issue in both ACNP and CNS education. While it is recognized by many that ACNPs and CNSs have different practice domains (Fenton & Brykczynski, 1993), the areas of overlap are obvious. A survey of graduate nursing programs in the United States (Forbes, Rafson, Spross, & Kozlowski, 1990) found marked similarities between the core curricula of CNS and NP programs. The only significant differences were that NP programs generally put a greater emphasis on pharmacology, primary care, physical assessment, health promotion, nutrition and history taking. This point is further supported by the results of a survey of CNS and NP graduates conducted in New York State ($n = 244$) which suggested that the differences found in practice are not as great as indicated in the literature (Elder & Bullough, 1990). While the role boundaries for APNs have been changing, there has been no clear direction for nursing education.

OTHER INFLUENCES

There is a broad range of external forces that are influencing the evolution of curricular standards for ACNP educational programs. These forces range from professional organizations and common practice to funding agencies and the results of evaluative efforts. Factors of specific importance are described below.

Professional Organizations

The two organizations that have provided the most significant direction to the evolution of the ACNP role have been the American Nurses Association and the American Association of Critical-Care Nurses. Although both organizations had done preliminary work independently in evaluating the growing need for APNs in direct care roles in acute care settings, they recognized the importance to the profession of collaborating to develop consensus regarding both scope of practice and certification.

American Association of Critical-Care Nurses (AACN)

In 1993, AACN formed an Advanced Practice Partnership to identify issues and reach consensus on assumptions about advanced practitioners and advanced practice (Caterinicchio, 1995). As an outgrowth of the Association's interest in advanced practice in critical care, an invitational conference was held in January 1994. At this conference, critical care leaders reaffirmed the Association's commitment to supporting the ACNP role and to working toward a consensus with the ANA to resolve questions about certification requirements.

American Nurses Association

In March of 1993, the American Nurses Association (ANA) Congress on Nursing Practice discussed the recent development of educational programs to prepare ACNPs and appointed an ACNP task force to be chaired by Dr. Jean Steel. In December 1993, the task force held its first face-to-face meeting and began drafting the "scope and standards." Input was sought on the draft using a nationwide field review. Once the input was available, the joint work group— composed of representatives from the ANA, the American Nurses Credentialing Center, the American Association of Critical-Care Nurses, and the AACN Certification Corporation—met and began work on a final document during the summer and fall of 1994. The end product of this collaborative effort is the *Scope of Practice for the Acute Care Nurse Practitioner and Standards of Clinical Practice for the Acute Care Nurse Practitioner* (American Association of Critical-Care Nurses and American Nurses Association, 1995).

TABLE 4.1   Key Elements of the ACNP Role

Clinical expertise
Integration of care across the acute care continuum
Establishment of processes for surveillance of care
Accountability and authority for patient outcomes across settings and
   boundaries
Evidence and research-based clinical practice
Advocacy/patient agency
Clinical leadership
Collaboration and coordination with all health care providers
Support of the design and management of systems which meet patients'
   needs
Adapability to changes within the role as patient/systems needs demand
Family assessment and discharge planning

Source: American Association of Critical-Care Nurses and American
Nurses Association. (1995). *Standards of clinical practice and scope of
practice for the acute care nurse practitioner.* Washington DC: American
Nurses Publishing.

   This document provides the basis for certified practice. Similar to
other scope documents, it delineates the profession's beliefs regarding the boundaries of practice, standards of performance, education,
and regulation of practice. The scope and standards also lay the
foundation for certification in professional practice. Key elements of
the ACNP role are listed in Table 4.1. The knowledge, skills, and
judgment that are outlined in the scope and standards form the basis
for the development of a certification exam (Kane, 1994; LaDuca,
1994).

American Association of Colleges of Nursing

The American Association of Colleges of Nursing (AACN) is an
organization that represents deans and directors of collegiate schools
of nursing. In March 1993, the membership approved a position
statement, *Nursing Education's Agenda for the 21st Century*
(AACN, 1993), that puts forth the role of nursing education in the
context of the ANA's *Nursing's Agenda for Health Care Reform.*
The position statement reviewed trends in health care and the na-

tional supply of nurses as well as providing guidelines for the future of nursing education. Among the trends particularly relevant for ACNP programs were a slight increase in total graduate school enrollments and an increasing prevalence of enrollments in graduate nursing programs for people with non-nursing backgrounds, as well as a projected shortfall of 200,000 in master's and doctorally prepared nurses by the year 2005 (American Association of Colleges of Nursing, 1993)

In addition, AACN has been particularly interested in advanced practice educational programs. It reviewed and made suggestions for the revision of NONPF's curriculum guidelines, and its 1994 conference focused on role differentiation of the nurse practitioner and Clinical Nurse Specialist. Reflecting the continued difference of opinion on this issue, an informal poll of participants at that conference revealed 68% to be in favor of merging the roles and 32% in opposition (American Association of Colleges of Nursing, 1995). Clearly this remains a topic for further discussion.

National Organization of Nurse Practitioner Faculties (NONPF)

As mentioned previously, the work of NONPF has been instrumental in guiding the development of many ACNP curricula. The National Organization is in the process of revising its *Nurse Practitioner Curriculum Guidelines* (Boodley, 1995). The specifics of these guidelines will continue to be important regardless of whether accrediting bodies, such as the National League for Nursing's Council on Baccalaureate and Higher Degree Programs, decide to formally endorse them.

Oncology Nursing Society

This is the first specialty nursing organization to have published advanced practice standards (Miaskowski & Rostad, 1990). In October 1994, the organization held the "ONS State of the Knowledge Conference on Advanced Practice" that included participants from the ONS, the Academy of Nurse Practitioners, the American Association of Critical-Care Nurses, the American Nurses Association, the Association of Pediatric Oncology Nurses, and the National League for Nursing. The recent findings of this conference have implications for curricula preparing APNs, including ACNPs, for oncology nursing.

Physician and Multidisciplinary Organizations

Members of several physician and multidisciplinary organizations are another potential source of influence. The American College of Cardiology held a consensus conference on the *Future Personnel Needs for Cardiovascular Health Care* (Gunnar & Williams, 1994), while the Society of Critical Care Medicine holds "controversy" sessions on the role of ACNPs in critical care at its annual meetings. Physician perceptions of ACNPs may be based more on their experience with other advanced practice nurses (midwives or anesthetists) than their experience with ACNPs, but their concerns and willingness to collaborate in practice are influential to role development.

Although physicians have actively participated in the development of ACNP programs across the country, there is an overall ambivalence about the role of ACNPs among physicians in general. Their concerns involve quality of care issues and patient outcomes, responsibility factors, degree of independent practice, and their own job security (Snyder et al., 1994). As American health care becomes more cost-efficient, there will be fewer positions for providers. And as APNs demonstrate their ability to manage complex patients in the acute care setting, they may replace physicians in some of these settings resulting in fewer positions being available to physicians, or, at the least, in increased competition for the remaining positions. This perceived competition for jobs, whether real or imagined, may influence the willingness of physicians to participate in or collaborate with ACNP programs in the future.

Funding Agencies

Agencies funding ACNP educational programs include the United States Public Health Service Division of Nursing, philanthropic foundations (Clochesy, Daly, Idemoto, Steel, & Fitzpatrick, 1994), and individual hospitals (Synder et al., 1994). These funding sources provide the opportunity to develop new programs and to influence the direction of curriculum development by selecting to fund those proposals that reflect particular approaches. The range of financial

TABLE 4.2 Examples of ACNP Programs Receiving External Funding by Source Type

Type of Funding Source	School/University
Hospital System	Case Western Reserve University
	University of Connecticut
Philanthropy/Foundation	Case Western Reserve University
Federal Training Grant	Rush University
	University of Kentucky
	University of Nebraska
	University of Pittsburgh
	University of South Carolina
	University of Southern Alabama

backing of ACNP programs demonstrates widespread support. A partial list of funded programs is shown in Table 4.2. Members of a growing network of professionals have been involved as consultants for many of the funded proposals.

Indirectly, funding agencies also influence educational standards further by supporting the evaluative phase of the training grants. This program evaluation and related research provides another key foundation for educational standards development. Research focused on evaluating the effectiveness and efficiency of the ACNP role affects educational directions in a similar, indirect fashion. Examples of such research include Mahoney's (1992) work on NPs as prescribers, Rudy and associates' work on the integration of mid-level practitioners into acute care hospitals (Rudy, Clochesy, Sereika, Davidson, & Daly, 1995), and Landefeld's (Genet et al., 1995; Landefeld, Rosenthal, & Brennan, 1992) randomized comparison of outcomes of NP care to house staff care.

STANDARDIZATION OF CURRICULUM CONTENT

Areas agreed upon at the first consensus conference that must be reflected in the ACNP curriculum include advanced assessment, advanced pathophysiology, pharmacology, diagnostic reasoning, clinical decision making, and advanced therapeutics (Standards for Educational Programs, 1993). While each of these areas may not have specific courses dedicated to them, it is essential that these areas be easily identifiable in course outlines and syllabi. Several of the following descriptions are further refinements of those included in the report of the 1993 consensus conference (Standards for Educational Programs, 1993), and are reflected in published reports of recently initiated ACNP programs (Clochesy, Daly, Idemoto, Steel, & Fitzpatrick, 1994; Hravnak et al., 1995; Keane & Richmond, 1993; Shah, Sullivan, Lattanzio, & Brutto-messo, 1993).

Advanced Assessment

Advanced assessment and differential diagnosis prepares a student to perform all aspects of health and illness assessment. These aspects include health history, risk appraisal, physical and mental status examination, selection of diagnostic studies and interpretation of the results, family assessment including social support systems, and evaluation of the home environment. Ideally, advanced assessment includes a clinical laboratory and precepted clinical experience.

Although advanced practice programs, such as CNS and primary care NP programs, have included assessment courses as part of the curriculum for some time, these same courses may not be sufficient for nurses whose practice will focus on acute illness and acute care settings. Faculty planning new ACNP programs need to evaluate the extent to which existing courses include adequate content on the identification and interpretation of abnormal findings and the use of diagnostic technology common in acute care, such as echocardiograms, ultrasounds, and ventilation/perfusion scans.

If additional assessment content is needed, there are three available approaches. The additional material can be incorporated into the existing assessment course. This is the simplest and least expensive alternative, but if a large majority of students in the course intend to practice in primary care areas, this may not be appropriate.

The additional content may then need to be provided to the ACNP students alone, either by offering a separate course (e.g., a 1- or 2-credit supplement to the standard assessment course) or incorporating this content into the clinical management courses.

Advanced Pathophysiology

Based on molecular biology and physiology, advanced pathophysiology provides a detailed study of the mechanisms of disease and provides the basis for nursing and medical management of patient problems. Pathophysiology is a basic clinical science that is common to all advanced practice students regardless of the population of interest or the practice setting. Currently, virtually all graduate programs require some physiology content in the curriculum and most programs can simply include the existing course in the ACNP program. However, if the existing course is more oriented toward normal physiology than abnormal, or if it is taught by nonclinical faculty from other schools, ACNP faculty may need to supplement the didactic material in the clinical courses with some discussion of specific disease mechanisms. Particularly important for part-time students, the pathophysiology course should be considered a prerequisite or at least co-requisite to the clinical courses.

Pharmacology

Pharmacology provides the knowledge that students need to prescribe medications and to assess patients' responses to pharmacologic therapy. This includes identification of individual and classes of drugs, their indications and contraindications, their likelihood of success, their side effects, and their interactions, as well as the laws and procedures governing writing prescriptions. Programs need to document 30–45 hours of pharmacology content to meet the prescriptive authority regulations in all jurisdictions. Because specific State Board regulations vary, it is wisest to plan on 45 hours to be certain the student will be able to practice in any state. At least one jurisdiction (the state of Washington) requires that the pharmacology course be taught in a School of Pharmacy.

Advanced Therapeutics/Clinical management

Advanced therapeutics provides the overall knowledge base for clinical practice. It integrates the information students gain in advanced assessment, advanced pathophysiology, and pharmacology with information about nonpharmacologic therapies and assessment of their effectiveness. This is an area with little standardization, but where much more work is needed. Most programs focus their attention on the cognitive skills needed by APNs in acute care. While this is important, others suggest that a set of procedural skills should be taught and competency expected of graduates. Clearly, both cognitive skills and procedural competencies belong in the clinical management courses and identifying effective teaching strategies present challenges to faculty.

The ability to integrate scientific knowledge and clinical observations in constructing hypotheses and a plan for confirming or rejecting the hypotheses is part of diagnostic reasoning (Carnevali, Mitchell, Woods, & Tanner, 1984). This is an essential cognitive skill for any practitioner who is going to be responsible for assessing and planning treatment regimens for patients and one of the most difficult skills for graduate students to learn. In addition to being a complex intellectual task, ACNP students are sometimes hampered by practice patterns learned as staff nurses and by the limitations imposed on advanced nursing practice by state regulations.

Most experienced staff nurses quickly learn the patterns and norms of practice at their institution and become quite knowledgeable about usual treatment approaches in their area of specialization. However, as staff nurses they have not had to assume responsibility for either creating these approaches or deciding in each individual case what modifications to the standard might be needed. Therefore, they often do not have an in-depth understanding of the rationale for the approach, the research findings on which treatment choices have been based, or the alternatives. Further, they are not accustomed to the responsibility of actually having to make these major treatment decisions prior to obtaining consultation, rather than contributing suggestions or offering critiques to someone else who bears final responsibility. Restrictive state regulations which prohibit acts of medical diagnosis by APNs or limit them to following established treatment protocols, with little leeway for individual judgment, also hamper nurses in learning. Thus, the acquisition of scientific knowledge necessary to support choices of therapy or diagnostic strategies, becoming adept at processing this information along with specific patient data, and becoming comfortable with the role of decision maker is a major step in the progression to advanced practice nurse.

A variety of teaching strategies can be useful in helping students learn the process of diagnostic reasoning. Most important of these is the opportunity to practice while in the student role. Activities such as patient rounds in the clinical setting in which students present their patients to other students and to ACNP faculty are excellent opportunities for students to attempt this process of synthesizing and concisely summarizing data, presenting diagnostic and treatment plans, and responding to questions that test his or her understanding. Writing their own treatment algorithms for specific conditions, including supporting rationale, is a good exercise for students early in the program. Use of computer-assisted technology programs, some of which have been designed for medical school use (e.g., the Med-CAPS programs), can also be appropriate teaching strategies. Although very few interactive video programs have as yet been designed for advanced practice students, this technology offers much promise for the future, and it will be important to work with vendors to design appropriate software.

When teaching procedural skills it is important to identify the level of competency expected and to plan the progression of skill acquisition and intensity of supervision by faculty and/or preceptors. Although students often are quite anxious about the need to acquire procedural skills, there are two reasons to be somewhat conservative in the number and variety of skills taught to all students. First, on a practical level, it is quite difficult in most settings to arrange adequate opportunities for learning many skills. Developing proficiency in these skills requires repeated practice by each student, under carefully chosen clinical conditions, and this often is not possible. For example, if we believed that all students should be able to perform lumbar punctures, each student should have at least three or four opportunities to perform the procedure. If there are 5 to 10 students in each class, 15 to 40 supervised lumbar punctures would be required. It is rather unlikely that these learning experiences can be provided. More important, one of the objectives for having an

ACNP as the primary care provider in the hospital is to move away from the practice of continually having novices providing most of the direct care. This dictates a philosophy that recognizes that today's health care provider cannot be expert in all areas and skills. Thus, ACNP students should be taught only those procedures that are likely to be relatively common in all settings and they should supplement their basic preparation with the acquisition of specific procedural skills common to their specialty once they have begun practice in a particular setting.

Clinical Experiences

The clinical practicum allows students the most valuable opportunity to integrate and synthesize knowledge about health and disease, research findings, and an advanced knowledge of pharmacology and therapeutics and to apply this knowledge to the needs of patients and their families. Issues that must be addressed include the appropriateness of settings for precepted clinical experiences, the necessary qualifications for preceptors, and the minimum amount of clinical experience.

Practice Settings

The *Scope of Practice* (AACN & ANA, 1995) states that the ACNP practices in *any* setting in which patient care requirements include complex monitoring and therapies, high-intensity nursing intervention, and continuous nursing vigilance. Therefore it would seem appropriate to apply these three criteria to potential clinical sites for students' precepted experiences. This raises the question of whether all student clinical experiences must take place in the inpatient setting, or whether outpatient settings could be used for some experiences such as physical assessment or physical diagnosis practicum. Other experiences needed by ACNP students may be more prevalent in a variety of specialized settings, either inpatient or outpatient, with both episodic and continuous patient care responsibilities.

Arguments in favor of the view that student experiences not be limited to inpatient settings include the suggestion to provide follow-through experiences for those students who are able to see their patients in clinics and offices after discharge. This affords them the opportunity to develop efficiency in performing rapid physical assessments and history taking. Additionally, proponents argue that outpatient settings are increasingly the site of most of health care, including acute care services that formerly were provided only in the hospital. Certainly some ACNPs will be practicing in both inpatient and outpatient settings after graduation and will want to obtain experience in both settings.

Although there are good reasons, as stated above, to include carefully selected outpatient experiences in the clinical practicum, the purpose of the role of the ACNP is to "provide advanced nursing care across the continuum of acute care services *to patients who are acutely and critically ill* (AACN and ANA, 1995)." The knowledge base to support this role cannot be obtained without devoting the majority of clinical time to caring for patients in acute care facilities.

Preceptors

Since the ACNP role is relatively new and it continues to evolve, it is difficult to identify a large number of ACNPs who are planning to serve as preceptors for students. Most often, a variety of preceptors are being used including other APNs, NPs and physicians. There are both advantages and disadvantages to using these non-ACNP preceptors. The most obvious limitation is that students do not observe ACNP practice as practiced by ACNPs. There has been a considerable discussion of the issues related to using physicians as preceptors for ACNP students. Physicians are excellent choices for differential diagnoses of diseases and for planning medical therapies. Further, physicians are good models of accountability in professional practice. Aside from the inability to model ACNP practice, physicians come from the medical-cure paradigm of health care delivery whereas APNs use a broader health restoration paradigm that includes, but is not limited to, the medical-cure model. Chapter 5 provides a more detailed discussion of the role of the nursing faculty member when working with physician preceptors.

Preceptor Qualifications

Preceptor selection requires a careful balancing of specialized knowledge (academic preparation) with clinical expertise (practice credentials). Further balancing is required between more structured experiences supervised by regular faculty and less structured experiences supervised by adjunct and clinical faculty. Regardless of choices, it seems reasonable to require that preceptors have a current practice involving the population in the same or a similar setting to the one in which they are precepting students.

Number of Students Supervised

The proposed revision of the NONPF *Nurse Practitioner Curriculum Guidelines* (Boodley, 1995b) goes beyond the curriculum to standards for faculty workload and faculty/student ratio. The proposal suggests:

> Supervision of all students in the clinical areas is the responsibility of nationally certified and practicing nurse practitioner program faculty. The maximum number of students that one NP program faculty supervises should not exceed six students in any one clinical course. If faculty are providing on-site clinical supervision of students, the maximum ratio is two students per faculty. If faculty are supervising students while managing their own caseload of patients, the maximum ratio is one student per faculty.

Minimum Clinical Experience

Ideally, the required clinical experience is whatever it would require to achieve the minimal clinical competencies of the program. In the absence of accepted competencies, a minimum of 600 clinical hours (Boodley, 1995b) is proposed. There is beginning evidence (Rogers, Grenvik, & Willenkin, 1995) that students can learn cognitive components of patient management skills using a format that encourages judgment, decision making, and analytic skills, despite the liabilities inherent to education in the complex, acute care setting. Rogers further demonstrated that such competencies can be measured.

At some future date, a list of competencies and methods for demonstrating achievement of the competencies should be developed. Once this is done, it would be more useful to talk about the median amount of time needed to achieve the competencies.

FACULTY QUALIFICATIONS

As advanced practice nursing evolves, emphasis will need to be put on the development of the expertise of faculty members. Initially, deans and program directors worry about having an adequate number of adequately credentialed (NP) faculty. This is only one aspect, albeit an immediate one, of the need for faculty development.

The curriculum dictates the expertise needed by faculty. Accrediting bodies require that faculty responsible for teaching the various courses at the university have adequate (graduate level) preparation in the areas that they are teaching. For example, the faculty member assigned to teaching pharmacology should have graduate preparation in pharmacology, preferably a graduate degree in the area. While this may seem unrealistic, it is common among universities to require documentation of a graduate faculty member's education, experience, and expertise in the area in which he or she is assigned to teach. The same is true for physiology, pathophysiology, and all other content areas. Many schools of nursing need to send faculty away for additional preparation and experience.

Planning for faculty members to obtain additional education to become nurse practitioners clearly requires a major commitment on the part of both the school and the individual. This is true regardless of whether faculty are freed from regular teaching responsibilities to travel out of state for the needed supplementary education or whether they must continue their regular teaching and research activities. There are several options for postmaster's APNs with acute care backgrounds. These include summer programs for postmaster's ACNP students, such as those offered at the University of South Carolina and the "executive practicum program" described by Jean Steel (chapter 2). The University of Colorado offers a postmaster's family NP program and the University of Wisconsin-Oshkosh offers a postdoctoral family NP program. The most important point in selecting a program is whether or not the course of study and faculty build on students' previous education and experience while preparing them for an increasing scope of practice.

The need to have faculty who have recent, if not current, practice experience is common to all NP programs. NONPF's Program Standards include the following among the faculty qualifications:

- Currently certified as a NP by a national certifying body
- maintaining currency in clinical practice, and
- meeting specialty requirements for continuing competency in accordance with their program responsibilities (Boodley, 1995b).

Although these standards were developed before the initiation of most ACNP programs, they represent a standard for which all new practitioner programs should aim. Consistent with this view, the American Nurses Credentialing Center's (ANCC) requirements for recertification for all nurse practitioner certifications, including ACNP, specify 1500 hours of clinical practice or direct clinical supervision (ANCCb, 1995) in each 5-year certification period.

To maintain clinical competency and to meet the recertification requirements, faculty must have time built into their schedules for practice. Regardless of whether this is done through the mechanism of a faculty practice plan, offering a nontenure track for faculty, or by simply recognizing clinical practice as part of the evaluation of faculty productivity, the faculty responsible for practitioner programs must have some mechanism that fosters the clinical component of their role.

It may be necessary, particularly in new programs, to use faculty from outside of the school of nursing to teach specific nonclinical classes, such as pathophysiology or pharmacology. In some instances, such a faculty member could be given a secondary appointment in the nursing school while maintaining his/her primary appointment in the academic department of expertise.

As health care becomes more complex, and the curriculum evolves to meet the needs of students and society, nursing faculties will need more expertise in basic or foundational support areas such as epidemiology, molecular biology, and pharmacology. To ensure a quality program, it is important that no program rely on the expertise of a single individual. Hence most deans and directors will need a long-term faculty development plan.

POINTS OF CONTINUING CONTROVERSY

As is typical of new roles and new educational programs, there are many aspects of ACNP education that remain unresolved. In addition to the debate regarding the merger of CNS and NP programs, discussed earlier, there is ongoing concern about the risk of producing a practitioner who is simply a replacement for house staff and functions solely in a medical model, as well as about questions related to the degree of clinical specialization.

The ACNP role is envisioned as situated in acute care facilities, where practice occurs in close collaboration with physicians. This necessarily means that the ACNP student must be prepared to function effectively within a system that is heavily organized around the medical model of disease-focused, episodic care. Faculty thus must assure that students are able to blend into existing practice routines, such as participating in clinical rounds, performing common technical procedures, documenting in a format that is understood by physician colleagues, and using consultants in a way that is familiar and acceptable to them. To reject all of these practical routines as belonging to the "medical model" is confusing simple aspects of the organizational culture of acute care facilities with the much more important aspects of nursing identity. At the same time, as nurse educators, we have a commitment to preparing APNs to function as nurses, with our traditional concern for holism, wellness, and continuity of care across organizational boundaries.

Students can be assisted to make the transition from staff nurse to APN by being expected, as students, to integrate risk assessment and discharge planning into their therapeutic regimens. They should be encouraged to propose health teaching and counseling approaches that will assist the patient in remaining well and out of the acute care setting. Formal examinations and other tests of knowledge base should include concepts from the behavioral and social sciences that are relevant to understanding the impact of illness on the patient and family.

The question of how much specialization is appropriate for incorporation into program plans is a familiar one in nursing education. It is particularly relevant in ACNP programs because many of these programs originated either in critical care programs or in response to the demand for practitioners in critical care settings. Factors that are important in addressing this question include the current approach to regulating practice. All states that recognize or regulate advanced practice through some sort of credentialing, whether that be a separate advanced practice license, a certificate, or a letter of recognition, are formally recognizing the practitioner's competency as a generalist, just as the RN license confirms beginning competency of the RN student in all areas of nursing. Thus, one can argue that the advanced practice credential should provide assurance to the public that the practitioner is prepared as a generalist. Specialty certification, such as has occurred with Family Nurse Practitioners and Gerontological Nurse Practitioners, becomes appropriate only when the knowledge base and practice become sufficiently diverse to support the development of specific competencies. Given the newness of the role of the ACNP and its educational programs, we are not yet ready as a profession to prepare and credential specialists within the general area of acute care.

The opposing view argues that advanced degree programs are, by definition, specialty focused. We have a long history of preparing nurses at the master's level in relatively narrow specialties, such as orthopedics, oncology, and cardiac critical care. In addition, some suggest that our knowledge base is already too wide to expect practitioners to be competent in all areas, and that advanced practice virtually necessitates some degree of specialization.

This issue is an important philosophical one that faculties should address before developing their curricula. It should also be noted that even if the generalist approach is chosen, this does not mean that programs cannot offer students opportunities to add specialty-focused content, such as critical care or oncology; however, this should be added to a solid foundational base of generalist preparation. Clearly, this means that such programs will be longer than those who do not offer this option. Some schools have incorporated a requirement for a full-time practicum in the student's last semester and used this as a time for the student to concentrate on those patient problems and management strategies common to the area in which he/she plans to work.

SUMMARY

Educational programs for ACNPs are a relatively recent development. There is general agreement among faculty about basic content areas. Evolving curricular and educational standards will be influenced for the foreseeable future by professional organizations and credentialing bodies, common practice, agencies funding training and research and the growing body of ACNP literature. Areas for standardization include the key curricular areas of advanced assessment, advanced pathophysiology, pharmacology, advanced therapeutics, and clinical experiences.

The key area for future development is process standards. Standards in this area will include faculty qualifications, clinical experiences, student supervision, and end-of-program competencies including procedural skills. Strategies for teaching diagnostic reasoning should be a continued focus for innovations. Unresolved issues that require further discussion include the possibility of merging the roles and preparation for CNS and ACNP, maintaining a strong nursing identity in the role of the latter, and balancing the need for specialty preparation with the expectation for competency as a generalist.

REFERENCES

American Association of Colleges of Nursing. (1993). *Nursing education's agenda for the 21st century*. Washington, DC: Author.

American Association of Colleges of Nursing. (1995). Proceedings of the Master's Education Conference. *Role differentiation of the nurse practitioner and clinical nurse specialist: Reaching toward consensus*. Washington, DC: Author.

American Association of Critical-Care Nurses and American Nurses Association. (1995). Scope of practice for the acute care nurse practitioner and standards of clinical practice for the acute care nurse practitioner. Washington, DC: American Nurses Publishing.

American Nurses Credentialing Center. (1995a). *1995 certification catalog*. Washington, DC: Author.

American Nurses Credentialing Center. (1995b). *1995 recertification catalog*. Washington, DC: Author.

Boodley, C. (1995a). Pew grant project. National Organization of Nurse Practitioner Faculties Executive Update, 4, 2.

Boodley, C. (1995b). Nurse practitioner educational guidelines: program standards, curriculum, and graduate outcomes. Proceedings of the Master's Education Conference. *Role differentiation of the nurse prac-*

titioner and clinical nurse specialist: Reaching toward consensus (pp. 59–68). Washington, DC: American Association of Colleges of Nursing.

Carnevali, D. C., Mitchell, P. H., Woods, N. F., & Tanner, C. A. (1984). *Diagnostic reasoning in nursing.* Philadelphia: J. B. Lippincott.

Caterinicchio, M. (1995). *Advanced nursing practice: Facts and strategies for regulation, reimbursement and prescriptive authority.* Aliso Viejo, CA: American Association of Critical-Care Nurses.

Clochesy, J. M., Daly, B. J., Idemoto, B. K., Steel, J., & Fitzpatrick, J. J. (1994). Preparing advanced practice nurses for acute care. *American Journal of Critical Care, 3,* 255–259.

Elder, R. G., & Bullough, B. (1990). Nurse practitioners and clinical nurse specialists: Are the roles merging. *Clinical Nurse Specialist, 4,* 78–84.

Fenton, M. V., & Brykczynski, K. A. (1993). Qualitative distinctions and similarities in the practice of clinical nurse specialists and nurse practitioners. *Journal of Professional Nursing, 9,* 313–326.

Forbes, K. E., Rafson, J., Spross, J. A., & Kozlowski, D. (1990). Clinical nurse specialist and nurse practitioner core curricula survey results. *Nurse Practitioner, 15*(4), 43–48.

Gawlinski, A., & Kern, L. S. (1994). *The clinical nurse specialist role in critical care.* Philadelphia: W. B. Saunders.

Genet, C. A., Brennan, P. F., Ibbotson-Wolff, S., Phelps, C., Rosenthal, G., Landefeld, C. S., & Daly, B. (1995). Nurse practitioners in a teaching hospital. *Nurse Practitioner, 20*(9), 47–54.

Gunnar, R. M., & Williams, R. G. (1994). 25th Bethesda Conference: Future Personnel Needs for Cardiovascular Health Care, *Journal of the American College of Cardiology, 24,* 275–328.

Hravnak, M., Kobert, S. N., Risco, K. G., Baldisseri, M., Hoffman, L. A., Clochesy, J. M., Rudy, E. B., & Snyder, S. V. (1995). Acute care nurse practitioner curriculum: Content and development process. *American Journal of Critical Care, 4,* 179–188.

Kane, M. T. (1994). Validating interpretive arguements for licensure and certification examinations. *Evaluation & the Health Professions, 17,* 133–159.

Keane, A., & Richmond, T. (1993). Tertiary nurse practitioners. *Image, 25,* 281–284.

LaDuca, A. (1994). Validation of professional licensure examinations. *Evaluation & the Health Professions, 17,* 178–197.

Landefeld, C. S., Rosentahl, G., & Brennan, P. F. (1992). A randomized trial of collaborative care: An alternative model for organizing health care delivery in teaching hospitals. Robert Wood Johnson Grant proposal, unpublished.

Mahoney, D. F. (1992). Nurse practitioners as prescribers: Past research trends and future study needs. *Nurse Practitioner, 17*(1), 46–51.

Mezey, M. (1993). Preparation for advanced practice. In M. Mezey & D. O. McGivern, *Nurses, nurse practitioners*, 2nd ed. New York: Springer Publishing Co., 31–58.

Miaskowski, C., & Rostad, M. (1990). *Standards of advanced practice in oncology nursing.* Pittsburgh, PA: The Oncology Nursing Press.

Rogers, P. L., Grenvik, A., & Willenkin, R. L. (1995). Teaching medical students complex cognitive skills in the intensive care unit. *Critical Care Medicine, 22,* 575–581.

Rudy, E. B., Clochesy, J. M., Sereika, S. M., Davidson, L. J., & Daly, B. J. (1995). *Integration of mid-level practitioners into acute care hospitals.* Robert Wood Johnson Foundation grant #023213.

Secretary's Committee to Study Extended Roles for Nurses. (1972). Extending the scope of nursing practice. *Nursing Outlook, 20,* 46–52.

Shah, H. S., Sullivan, D. T., Lattanzio, J., & Bruttomesso, K. M. (1993). Preparing acute care nurse practitioners at the University of Connecticut. *AACN Clinical Issues in Critical Care Nursing, 4,* 625–629.

Snyder, J. V., Sirio, C. A., Angus, D. C., Hravnak, M. T., Kobert, S. N., Sinz, E. H., & Rudy, E. B. (1994). Trial of nurse practitioners in intensive care. *New Horizons, 2,* 296–304.

Standards for educational programs: Preparing students as acute care nurse practitioners. (1993). *AACN Clinical Issues in Critical Care Nursing, 4,* 593–598.

Zimmer, P. A., Brykczynski, K., Martin, A. C., Newberry, Y. G., Price, M. J., & Warren, B. (1990). *Advanced nursing practice: Nurse practitioner curriculum guidelines.* Seattle, WA: National Organization of Nurse Practitioner Faculties.

Chapter 5

ACQUIRING CLINICAL SKILLS AND INTEGRATING THEM INTO THE PRACTICE SETTING

Helen S. Shah, DNSc, RN

At least one element will remain constant as the profession elaborates the ideal preparation of an acute care nurse practitioner (ACNP): clinical experience. Programs need to include a sufficient clinical base to make the ACNP a valuable, contributing, and reliable partner in the care delivery team. What form the clinical component will eventually take and which minimal expectations will be invoked remain to be seen. What is currently true is that the path from the drawing boards of faculty and curriculum meetings to the actual clinical bedside is not straightforward. The following chapter describes some of the issues involved in planning for student arrangements in the clinical area and issues that might challenge their success during the program of study as well as after its completion.

PRELIMINARY PLACEMENT ARRANGEMENTS

Contracting with Preceptors

In most graduate nursing education programs faculty negotiate clinical experience by contacting the nursing preceptors who will become involved with the respective students. This is often through direct communication with the persons themselves. Alternatively, the nursing education office of the target hospital provides the coordination of student and preceptor matches, limiting access to a particular preceptor by too many students or faculty (Shah & Polifroni, 1992). In either situation, the nursing education department serves as a buffer for student guests, providing logistical and safety orientation to the agency.

Arrangements for the ACNP clinical experience take several forms. In some cases the preceptor may be a traditional clinical nurse specialist (CNS) while other cases demand the presence of physicians. Nurse practitioners may also serve as preceptors. This new role preparation demands elements of preceptorship expertise that reside in more than one individual. It is important for the faculty member to understand the types of clinical practice potential that preceptors have.

Advanced Practice Nurse Preceptors

In some instances traditional CNSs have direct care responsibility and accountability. Some are affiliated with multispecialty medical practice groups and may or may not be employees of the host institution. These APNs provide care for patients of the entire group, depending on their own specialty orientation. Others, employed in hospitals, have been able to create strong practice bases within their settings. Some CNSs may also have prescriptive authority for medications and diagnostic testing. Others have developed their practices with primary responsibilities to the nursing staff and indirect patient care responsibilities. Often they have research or educational obligations and represent their specialty or patient units at hospital departmental committees. They serve as consultants to a wider scope of colleagues and activities while performing fewer bedside clinical functions. Primary care nurse practitioners (NPs) also are a rich source for preceptor experiences. Engaging in diagnostic reasoning processes with management responsibilities for their patients, NPs can help ACNP students learn those elements of practice. Both types of APNs, CNSs and NPs, have much to contribute to the development of the students.

Physician Preceptors

If APNs are insufficient in number or type of practice, physicians are often willing to assist ACNP students. In physician practices specialization shapes the parameters as well as the location of their practices. Those physicians whose practice is office based do not spend great amounts of time in the hospital visiting their patients. While they are able to teach students diagnostic reasoning, management of their patients occurs primarily in community settings.

Of those physicians who are hospital based, some function in administrative capacities and have limited direct care responsibilities while others spend all of their time in direct patient care. It is often the former who are involved in negotiating student placement, so it is important for them to articulate the needs and abilities of the students with the preceptors who will be directly involved. Close attention to medical specialties is also in order. Surgical practitioners spend much time performing surgical procedures. Unless it is the intention of the program or the ACNP student to develop a perioperative focus, this is not a recommended match. It is the management of the care and not necessarily the procedures that need attention.

Faculty Role

As with conventional arrangements for graduate students, the faculty member contacts the preceptor directly and negotiates activities and scheduling. Additional detail regarding objectives, expectations, and curriculum should be provided as the preceptor is most likely prepared for a different type of role (CNS or other type of NP). This negotiation needs to be more comprehensive with physicians than is usually the case with nurse colleagues. The physician preceptors may or may not be aware of the ACNP role. Even if they are, they may not have had any experience with ACNPs. Regardless of awareness and experience, physician preceptors share similar backgrounds in their own training that have implications for their work with nursing students. They not only need briefing on the goals of the experience and the abilities of the students but also on the expectations of how they will effect students' learning.

Contact for physician preceptors, as with nurse preceptors, may be made directly with a preceptor or through the medical faculty, depending on the facility. Full-time clinical directors are often easier to contact and can facilitate arrangements for students by assuming responsibilities themselves or negotiating for others to do so. When more than one clinical service is involved, as is often the case, the contact is more readily made with the dean/associate dean or the chief-of-staff as well as the chief-of-service. On less frequent occasions, the contact may be initiated by the preceptor. Physicians who have previously collaborated with nurse practitioners and value their contributions sometimes wish to participate in their education. Rare and potentially valuable resources like these need encouragement and support to overcome any system barriers that may be present.

The importance of maintaining contact with the nursing education department when working with physician preceptors does not change. Logistics regarding identification badges, health and licensure screening, safety and physical plant orientation remain vital. An additional courtesy is to extend pertinent information regarding the proposed clinical activity to the management and CNS staff of the affected clinical units.

Schedule Conflicts

An essential element present in the practitioner role not usually found in other types of nursing care providers is the concept of continuity of responsibility. This concept is not a new one to nursing. When primary nursing was introduced as a vehicle for increasing patient and nurse satisfaction with care, it promised to reflect this element. The primary nurse was to have 24-hour responsibility for patient care, delegated to another nurse when off shift. In reality, however, shortages of professional nurses and multiple, complex scheduling schemes soon prohibited this aspiration (Phipps, Cassmeyer, Sands, & Lehman, 1995). Even at its peak, primary care responsibility did not resemble the same continuous responsibility practitioners are required to develop for their patients. Nurses' roles have usually permitted them to be on duty or off duty as the schedule dictates. While off duty, patient responsibility ends unless the individual has on-call accountability. Of the several types of APNs, traditional CNSs have limited continuous patient responsibility because the majority of them do not assume primary nurse roles.

The net result is a clash between the expectation of the students entering a graduate program and their need for learning to provide practitioner care. Many students are part-time and juggle the demands of family and work to accommodate academic activities. At great personal sacrifice, many have learned to manipulate their work time to extended weekend "supershifts" or package their vacation time with holidays. Thus they create pockets of time available for their clinical responsibilities. For the traditional CNS role, this is a successful strategy. Even for the primary care practitioner role, the episodic nature of patient care permits this type of flexible scheduling.

These calendar acrobatics fail when it comes to the ACNP role, however. Patients in the acute phase of their illnesses, hospitalized and very ill, require vigilance throughout the period of hospitalization. Medications, tests, and treatments ordered on one day require evaluation of results on the next day or perhaps even sooner. The care team orchestrates most activity for patient care in the main part of the day during patient rounds. While adjustments are frequently necessary later in the day, they do not constitute the main phase of clinical planning. To become an accepted part of the team, the practitioner has to participate in patient rounds. These occur daily while the patient remains in the hospital. To schedule participation in a daily event on an episodic basis distorts its value and leads to frustration of the team members as well as the student. Consequently the clinical practicum must include consecutive days of clinical experience. Prospective students must be informed of this expectation before beginning the program so that they can make appropriate arrangements of their schedule.

Clinical Practicum Location

Another aspect of the educational program that will need to be addressed in planning to initiate an ACNP clinical course concerns the relationship the student enjoys with the respective placement hospital. When the goals of preparation for CNSs are consultation, leadership, and education for the indirect care-giving role, placement at their own hospitals has many disadvantages for students. If students remain in their own hospitals, they take advantage of their informal networks to accomplish their tasks. They already know the strengths and weaknesses of members of the nursing staff on their units and often on other units as well. They also often know members of the care delivery team from other departments including social services, nutritional services, pharmacy, pastoral care, and medicine.

This apparent advantage is, in reality, a crutch. The art of consultation is one to be learned, not commandeered by virtue of position nor intuited with personal knowledge. When students are assigned to agencies other than their own, the leadership and consultative attributes of their preceptors can be better analyzed and emulated.

For ACNP students the situation is somewhat different. When the goal of practitioner preparation is to produce strong and competent direct care providers, certain advantages exist in the placement of individuals within their own practice setting, albeit in a new role. The practitioner is already familiar with the present systems operation as well as with many of the other members of the health care team. Priority is direct care that is safe, efficient, cost-effective, and holistic. The knowledge of other members of the care team is vital and permits more efficiency in learning diagnostic reasoning and patient care management. Former colleagues are a source of support to the students in a new role. The students do not need to learn how to get things done for patients, but rather what things need doing. This degree of stability is desirable in the tumultuous road to becoming a practitioner.

Occasionally a situation may arise when it is not in the best interest of the student to be reassigned to a current work setting. Reasons vary but may involve the relationship of the student to the agency and the vision of the administrators. If the student is perceived by the unit manager or supervisors as ill chosen for the new role, the needed support will be lacking. And if the vision of the agency involves deploying only practitioners with previous experience within other advanced practice roles, expectations will be too high for the student to succeed. These variables underscore the need for the faculty member to learn as much as possible about the hospital and all key players in the educational process there.

Work-study options represent another placement arrangement for innovative nursing and hospital administrators. If the agency considers permitting the student to remain an employee (in a training/orientation mode for salary purposes) and the school agrees to credit this clinical experience, a work-study type of program can result. Naturally, the objectives and curricular needs of the program have to be respected by the agency. The benefits from this type of arrangement accrue to students, hospitals, and schools.

The advantage to the students is that some degree of gainful employment persists throughout the educational period, including the time with intense clinical demands. In view of the difficulty students encounter financing their education, this is a vital point. A less tangible advantage is the degree of comfort the students perceive in remaining at their own base.

The gain to the agency is that a valuable employee is not lost while fulfilling educational requirements. The agency in effect is producing a highly desirable type of practitioner with mastery of its own system idiosyncrasies, thus saving the orientation period usually necessary for newly hired personnel. Furthermore, the student who has completed the program is motivated to remain with the institution in the new role rather than looking elsewhere for a position. Legal advantages may also be present when the student remains an employee. Employee status can facilitate risk management while student status often complicates it. Hospital administrators may prefer practitioner students to be employees rather than visitors to avoid potential legal complications in this period of role evolution.

Faculty also realize an advantage in work-study arrangements. Placement is facilitated with the hospital administrators and student employees taking such an active role, identifying potential preceptors and clinical units for experiences. However, a certain degree of diplomacy is needed by the faculty in initiating such arrangements. Not all hospitals are prepared to launch this new type of practitioner within their confines. In some cases, the nursing administrators embrace the concept but the medical department places varying obstacles in their way. The converse is also possible. The faculty member must be willing to provide the necessary information to effect new opportunities: explanation of the new role, how it has been successful, any known problems, and referral to other successful sites. Often many meetings are required involving all representatives from all disciplines.

To begin any placement process it is important to identify an innovative administrator with whom to dialogue. If the person is highly placed within the institution, the managers and clinicians who will be affected need to be included in the early meetings as well. Concerns of nursing administrators usually involve reporting structures, scheduling, and relationships to the nursing and medical staffs. Concerns of the medical department members usually include competing demands of medical students, malpractice liability and the actual responsibility for patients. Within the medical hierarchy responsibilities are differentially distributed among the different levels of house staff and attending physicians. The medical department has the need to know where on this distribution list the NP would fit. The challenge for the faculty member is to try to explain the ACNP role with few, if any, examples extant and to also understand the hierarchical arrangements within the individual agency. The subtle and often unspoken assumptions of medical practitioners' ascendancy of authority require faculty to use diplomacy and have a clear vision to explain the new hospital order and the role of the ACNPs within it.

Clinical Competition

An additional consideration of student status is noteworthy. Hospitals are fertile learning environments for many types of students, not only nursing. The ACNP role demands learning activities in many areas of the hospital, such as the emergency room, the operating room, and radiology. These areas are visited by many other types of students, including nurse anesthetists, medical students, physician assistants, and technical program students such as radiology technicians, emergency medical technicians, and surgical assistants. The question arises at times as to whose learning needs should have priority in certain situations, particularly if procedures are involved. Do physicians in training automatically receive priority in all situations? Delicate negotiations are required to forestall frustration. Experience indicates that the discipline of the preceptor (nurse or physician) influences the degree of preference for student learning.

Nurses tend to be comfortable with nursing students, nurse anesthetists with nurse anesthetist students, physicians with medical students, and so forth.

A successful method for diffusing this potential problem resides in the preceptor. Most preceptors, nurse or physician, are committed to their charge and relish the experience of creating another skilled practitioner. They make elaborate arrangements with their colleagues for assistance in other clinical areas where they do not themselves practice (e.g., the intensive care units and operating room). Nurse preceptors have long been sensitive to the learning competition. Physicians, though, are often unaware of the priority given to students other than their own, particularly in situations where they are not present. Careful and explicit discussions regarding this problem in advance of the learning period helps to avoid it. Simple solutions may involve only rescheduling while other situations may need verbal exploration and values clarification. Permission to champion the cause of the student is often all that is required for the preceptor to accept the challenge and guarantee the student's learning needs.

PHYSICIAN COLLABORATION

Traditionally, preceptors for advanced graduate work in nursing have been other advanced graduate nurses. For ACNP students this is a serious problem. Although there are individual exceptions and specialty considerations, nurses already in advanced practice within acute care settings (CNSs) do not implement their roles as primary providers of direct care. This creates a lack of adequate preceptor models for ACNPs. This situation is not unique to acute care however. When the early move to practitioner roles started, there were no NPs. In the beginning of the nurse anesthetist practitioner movement, the preceptors needed were physicians (Gunn, 1983; Silver, Ford, & Day, 1968). The same situation is present in the move to ACNP. The need to use physicians as clinical preceptors has several implications for nursing faculty responsible for these courses.

TABLE 5.1 Educational Considerations for Physician Preceptors

Difference	Description	Action
Aculturization	Learning takes priority over all else through total immersion in clinical arena.	Preclinical discussion and arrangements
Pedagogy	Teaching/learning based on extemporaneous and detailed elucidation of scientific supporting data.	Alternative teaching methods in pre clinical and clinical courses; practice sessions in classroom.
Cloak of responsibility	Decision making is discomforting when immediate action is required.	Build practitioner confidence gradually and seek preceptor assistance.

Educational Differences

When using physicians as preceptors for ACNP students, it is essential that nursing faculty be aware of the differences between traditional physician education and nursing education. These differences, outlined in Table 5.1, have implications for discussions with physician preceptors and for preparation of students for working with their preceptors.

Aculturization

The first difference between typical physician and nurse educational systems is the aculturalization that occurs in medical education with respect to the time of the student. Physicians in training spend all of their time at clinical activities. If an unplanned event occurs, it is not unusual for the physician to remain in place until it is settled.

If impromptu learning is required with the students' preceptors (attendings, senior-ranked residents and fellows), a conference room nearby is simply appropriated and informal class held. Scheduled conferences are frequently postponed or rescheduled as patient-care needs dictate. The net result is that physicians in training spend a great deal of both scheduled and unscheduled time on site, maximizing their learning.

For nurses, this becomes a source of frustration. Nursing education, even if done full time, is often superimposed upon other conflicting responsibilities of work and family. Preceptors who are accustomed to the medical education format are puzzled by that of nursing. In their enthusiasm for teaching and student learning, they regard any fractured attention to clinical learning as a reduction in commitment on the part of the student. This places unnecessary barriers in the relationship of student and mentor.

Preceptors must be helped to understand the nuances of the difference between nursing students and physician students. House officers can easily arrange for released time or coverage of their patients with colleagues. Nurse practitioner students electing to spend the extra time in the clinical arena may not be able to make up the missing segment with coverage or release. Their schedules may not be fully within their control. Nursing systems are not overly permissive for compensatory time. Furthermore, there may not be sufficient practitioners available with whom to arrange coverage. To avoid these conflicts, full exploration of the problems should be accomplished before the start of the clinical learning period.

Pedagogy

Another problem is pedagogical. Quite simply, nursing faculty methods of teaching are very different from those of physician faculty. For physicians much learning occurs on patient rounds when unanticipated questions are raised and participants are expected not only to know the answers but raise the questions within the group. Furthermore, they are expected to elucidate the problem with physiological and pathological detail until they have convinced their listeners about their own critical thinking and conclusion, all the while maintaining a certain rapid tempo. Active participation in this activity is a humbling process that strikes fear into the heart and soul of every student, medical and nursing alike. Physicians quickly learn mechanisms to succeed. Nurses will also, given a firm foundation in the supporting sciences. Yet this learning has few parallels in nursing and this situation can create discouragement. This is particularly true for postmaster's students who are accustomed to commanding respect and having the answers to questions. Therefore, it is imperative to change the methods used in graduate classrooms to a problem-based learning format.

Students must be provided the opportunity in the classroom to practice behaviors that will be expected in the clinical setting. This usually involves presenting patient situations and care plans in very concise, organized frameworks and responding extemporaneously to questions and suggestions from others. Students learn from each other by identifying what needs to be known about a problem, what is known, what can help, what has or has not worked in the past and why, and what will need to be done for resolution. The safety of the classroom provides the stage upon which students can develop the skills for thinking aloud, for recognizing errors in judgements, responding to peer criticism, and using probabilistic clinical reasoning (Don, 1994; Manning, Olmesdahe, Philpott, Friedman, & Loening, 1994; Trevitt & Grealish, 1994).

Responsibility

The third problem is more abstract. Nurses have learned to excel at providing quality nursing care. They often contribute essential assessment findings to confirm a diagnosis or wisely interpret technical data to avert clinical disasters. Nurses create complementary data bases for their patients upon admission that are frequently the source of information recorded by the physician in the history and physical examination. On many patient units, nurses are integral components of the care team and participate in the information sharing and decision making for their patients. Frequently there is a certain amount of second guessing that nurses share over shift reports and meal breaks. All of this occurs within a specific chain of command and much of it is based on retrospective views of the clinical course of patients. When NPs have to take the lead in creating the data base, supplement it with appropriate laboratory and imaging tests, confirm diagnostic reasoning and plan accordingly, a not-so-subtle shift in responsibility occurs. Donning the cloak of responsibility, albeit in collaboration with others, simply feels different. Even packaging the information for a coherent and comprehensive presentation of the patient is new. Primary care NPs have known this for years. Acute care nurse practitioners are beginning to learn, but physician preceptors may assume they come to the clinical situation comfortable with this responsibility.

Based on the existing differences, it is imperative to have thoughtful, planned discussions with the physician preceptors. The following negotiation points will be helpful for both nurse and physician preceptors but particularly for the latter.

An explanation that the preceptor will be viewed to some extent as a mentor or sponsor is a good beginning. Full disclosure of what exactly is meant by that is recommended (Hayes & Harrell, 1994). Preceptors teach the way they were taught and physician education is unlike that for nurses. Whereas nurses have had preceptors and somewhat fixed structures for learning, physicians were drawn into the learning environment with the assistance of the more senior house staff, often changing services frequently and not depending on any particular individual. A one-to-one ratio of student to mentor is a new experience for some.

The preceptor and student will be assessing individual learning needs together. The preceptor hopefully will facilitate the student's participation in learning activities planned for other students such as special rounds, grand rounds, skill development, noon conferences, etc. The preceptor should offer assistance with skill development or at least know that this is an expectation. Any specific competencies desired by the students require identification by them. Most students differ in previous experience or opportunity so that individual competencies vary. Agreement on the evaluation methods should be clarified. If weekly progress checks are needed with the student, both the preceptor and student should know this and set up a mechanism for these checks. If frequent updates and reality checks are to be given to the faculty, these need to be articulated.

A preliminary meeting, before the beginning of the practicum, is needed to discuss the culture of the institution and any expectations of behavior and dress. Scheduling and identification of additional teaching staff take place at this time. Introductions to key team members are useful as well; this would include fellows, residents at different postgraduate levels, physician assistants, clinical nurse specialists, division directors, and nurse managers.

The bulk of the clinical work involves sharpening assessment and judgment abilities and moving along a continuum of initial assessment to progressive case management to personal case load, as illustrated below:

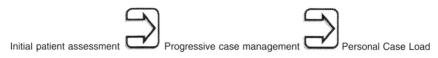

Initial patient assessment   Progressive case management   Personal Case Load

FIGURE 5.1   Continuum of ACNP Role Development.

Facilitating the students' learning in other departments such as radiology, anatomic and tissue pathology, or cardiology is a preceptor expectation. This includes identification of the designated persons at the other departments who will facilitate the students' learning. In some instances this person might be an administrative department head but an individual clinical practitioner usually works best. Seeing to these details presumes interest in teaching on both the part of the preceptor and preceptor designate.

Another difference in educational expectations between nurses and physicians pertains to the practitioner. Psychomotor skills are generally handled differently within medical education. The "see one, do one, teach one" approach contrasts to the more methodical progression from the review of procedure manuals to the classroom/ clinical laboratory approach. Many skills are gained through observing the more experienced practitioner. Unlike the pattern of nursing education in which nursing faculty are involved with the classroom laboratory teaching and accompany students to the patient bedside for initial procedures, physicians in training may prevail upon more senior house staff to assist them in skill acquisition. An individual preceptor will most likely delegate responsibilities for procedures to the team or individuals responsible for their performance. This person may be another physician, a CNS, an NP, or a PA.

Expectation for skill acquisition is an important item for students as well. They need to know the importance of learning only those things that will become a routine part of their practice. Students often focus on the need to learn procedures and they need to be reassured that, in most situations, procedures constitute a relatively small portion of practice. More emphasis should be placed on the management of patients within a holistic philosophy of care, knowing that procedures can also be learned as needed at a future time.

Preceptors also need to learn of the faculty member's own expectations. Occasional visits to the clinical site are necessary for full student evaluation despite the burden this places on the team by the presence of additional people. The faculty needs to know which members of the clinical staff participate in the students' learning experiences. Strong relationships forged through ongoing collaboration permit frank discussions of student abilities. Preceptors also have much to contribute regarding program design and revision.

Preceptor Types

There are generally four types of physician preceptors within hospitals depending on their size and structure. Full-time attendings are desirable preceptors by virtue of the fact that they are full-time at that institution. Visiting attendings may have admitting privileges at more than one agency and therefore may split their time and attention among several sites, including their nonhospital affiliated office or clinic. While visiting attendings may be enthusiastic and willing preceptors, creative planning will be required for a successful experience.

House staff or fellows and postgraduate officers are persons in training. As described by Benner (1984) novice teachers are often highly effective with novice learners as they have so recently been associated with that status. House staff commiserate with students and generally are eager to assist in their learning. Full-time attendings may assign one resident or fellow the responsibility of teaching the nurse practitioner, resulting in positive experiences for both.

Medical students present a source of surprise and pride. Familiarity with clinical situations, medications, treatment modalities, and institutional operations on the part of ACNPs increases their self-esteem when assisting medical students. While some nurses have viewed medical students with disdain and attribute to them a degree of ignorance of the situation at hand, NPs soon realize that medical students have much to offer. Nurse practitioner students are often surprised at the extent of the knowledge of foundational sciences that medical students have. It is fortuitous when each can offer the other assistance.

In an ideal world, nursing students learn from nursing practitioners. However, the real world offers both opportunities and the necessity to have them work with physician preceptors. Individual differences exist and there are many types and levels of physicians within institutions. The most successful formula for physician preceptors is a committed attending physician who loves to teach and is in a position within the hospital to provide or arrange for immediate supervision of the practitioner student within the unit setting and in supplementary departments.

INTEGRATION INTO EXISTING SYSTEMS

It is helpful when attempting to insert NPs into a given system if other NPs already exist somewhere within that system, e.g., neonatal or clinic practitioners. When this is not the case, decisions need to be made about where the ACNP will fit with respect to other advanced positions within the organization. For institutions, the ACNP is a guarantor of quality and unfragmented care, and can thus be viewed as an investment. As with any position, a job description, credentialing guidelines, and performance evaluation expectations are essential. These aspects, discussed in more detail in chapter 6, have some implications for the educator placing students in the setting and planning curricula.

Assumptions of the role

Utilization

It may be obvious in settings in which different types of practitioners already exist but utilization of NPs will differ according to their area of specialization. For example, in a critical care unit, the practitioners will be located primarily on the unit itself with all its attendant quirks for staff coverage. A cardiology NP, on the other hand, may have responsibilities within the coronary/critical care unit but also on the step-down and general medical units. Responsibilities may even extend to the outpatient unit, depending on the agency. The result is a broad geography of coverage.

Faculty need to know about this distribution before placing students within those settings. The schedules kept by the NPs may not be compatible with the academic schedule required of the student. For example, the best learning clinic opportunity may occur at a time when classes are meeting. There is also a potential for an overlapping of student experiences when students are assigned to different individual preceptors but end up together because the patients are shared among services.

Collaboration

It is imperative that everyone understand the collaborative nature of the ACNP and physician patient management. Neither is excluded from the decision-making process; a rather collegial agreement is the goal in making care decisions. Any deviation from the plan of care is carefully considered by the ACNP in view of usual and customary practice, prevailing scientific opinion, and predetermined accord. As with any care decision, the plan is seldom made in a vacuum. To the extent that the ACNP is practicing advanced nursing independently, within the legal and professional scope of practice, decisions made are subject to review and reinterpretation by other professionals on the care delivery team.

The transition to this type of practice is based on a clear under-standing by the NPs of the meaning of collaboration. They may even have to articulate this understanding to their physician colleagues. The challenge for the faculty member is to assure that students are launched on this transition with the knowledge and skill required for collaboration. Mature students and those who have had previous advanced practice roles accomplish this with greater ease. This has implications for student admissions and selection and for curriculum content. Assistance with role development is an essential ingredient that should be included in programs of study.

Focus of Practice

This assumption refers to the premise that ACNPs are not primarily physician substitutes nor assistants to physicians. As nurses they give primacy to holistic approaches to patients that include family and other support structures. Any practice pattern that places a greater emphasis on procedures and other technical skills is not consistent with the philosophy underlying the education of the ACNP.

Some potential ACNP students who practice at the bedside and wish to achieve advanced practice standing and prescriptive authority only view performance of procedures done and the order writing as evidence of advanced practice. In this regard they are similar to early undergraduate students who are only able to view nursing through the lens of tasks accomplished. Initially, graduate students may share this focus on procedural skills and will have to broaden their understanding of the meaning of advanced practice. Nursing faculty will have to assist these students to look beyond procedures and change their understanding so that they will be positioned to help others do likewise.

Schedule

The work schedule of ACNPs reflects their membership on the health care team. While everyone acknowledges that patient care is continuous throughout the day, it is clear that the majority of planning occurs during weekdays and day hours. Viewing the ACNP role as a method for coverage of off-shift time and areas of resident physician shortage is short-sighted and antithetical to the purpose of the role. Students should be given the skills needed to negotiate for job placement so that they are not placed in positions where their contributions are of limited value. This refers to type of patient case load as well as time of day.

Dual Reporting

This last assumption refers to the reporting and evaluative structure for the ACNP role. Ideally, the ACNP reports to both a nurse as well as a physician. The nursing department is justified in keeping control over the practitioner positions for reasons of finance but also because this role is a nursing role. Nursing is the familiar grounding for the ACNP and can provide a certain degree of comfort and network potential. On the other hand, nursing supervisors are hard pressed to offer clinical performance evaluation because of their own unfamiliarity with this type of practice. For this clinical judgment, performance review should come from those involved with the clinical decisions being made—usually, the medical staff. This requires strong collaborative arrangements among the nursing and medical administrators as well.

Faculty who have collaborative relationships with hospitals can contribute to this by helping both sides see the value and necessity of these arrangements. If joint appointments already exist between departments or between the school and the hospital, they can serve as models for the new role's placement within the organizational structure.

Job Description

The job description generally includes a description of the responsibilities of the position, the reporting structure, and qualifications. Language reflecting the direct delivery of advanced practice nursing is indicated. Specification of the kind of activities involving the participation in and management of patient care that distinguish this role from that of other APNs is also important. At times job descriptions reflect broad-brush descriptions of the actual work to be done. Exact details of function are deliberately omitted. Identification of the individuals who will be evaluating the ACNP's performance can provide additional indications of the type of role envisioned.

Expectations of academic and clinical preparation is important to prevent confusion. Recent use of the term *case management* has proliferated. The label applies to advanced practice roles only some of the time. Instances abound of designated case managers who are not prepared at the postbaccalaureate level of education. It is imperative to attain compatibility between the job candidates' abilities and education and the agency expectations.

Faculty assist students by including content in the curriculum that assesses several model job descriptions before the completion of the program of study. Advantages and disadvantages can be analyzed and strategies developed to assure maximum compatibility for the students.

Credentialing

Credentialing is a process through which an individual is ascertained to be properly educated, trained, certified, and licensed to provide services within an institutional setting. Authority for the institutional credentialing process may reside with the hospital administration, its medical staff, the board of trustees or any combination of the above. The process also involves an award of privileges to perform specific services within an institution. These privileges are often controlled through the hospital's medical staff. Credentialing should be re-evaluated at specific yearly intervals (Joint Commission on Accreditation of Hospitals, 1995).

Credentialing of nurses beyond state registration to work in hospitals is rare. In the past, except for nurse anesthetists and nurse midwives, only those individuals with highly specialized practices, such as enterostomal therapists, were expected to apply for hospital credentials. In the future, ACNPs will be expected to be properly credentialed within their institutions. The match between the practitioners' abilities and the institutions' needs requires vigilance to assure that only those practitioners educated to care for acutely ill patients are permitted to practice within those settings. Suitable credentialing methods for ACNPs are still in the evolutionary phase.

Dual service credentialing is recommended. For the nursing service, appropriate safeguards to ensure valid licensing and preparation already exist. For physicians, a similar safeguard is in place in the form of the medical staff credentialing committee or privilege control oversight committee. Patient safety is assured when only those individuals capable of providing the necessary care are permitted to do so. With ACNP roles, the medical staff have a vested interest in guaranteeing that the practitioners have received adequate clinical training before establishing collaborative patient care delivery. This necessitates meticulous record keeping on the part of the ACNPs before initiating employment as well as for ongoing development and reemployment.

Faculty should encourage students to chronicle all their clinical activities. The types of patients treated, experience with procedures, different patient units covered, individuals who have served as preceptors, and any additional descriptive information regarding practice may be examined by reviewing committees.

Performance Evaluation

If the reporting structure is shared by the nursing and medical departments, the evaluation originates with each. As described above, few nurse managers are able to evaluate the specifics of patient care delivery. However, they are able to evaluate the ACNPs' contribution to the nursing milieu of the involved units. Collaboration with other nurses, responding to their consultative requests, facilitating their educational needs, supporting research activities, and participating in unit-problem solving are only a few of the areas where a nursing supervisor would have more influence. On the other hand, medication type, dosing decisions and treatment adjustments based on laboratory findings are within the purview of a physician supervisor.

RELATIONSHIPS TO OTHER HEALTH CARE TEAM MEMBERS

The ACNP is focused on providing direct patient care but this cannot be done alone. Many other members of the care team come into contact with ACNPs and it is important that they all understand this new role. The more recognition there is of each member's special contribution, the better and more efficient will be the flow of care.

Nurse/Unit Managers

Nurse managers and ACNPs enjoy a relationship parallel to that between the manager and CNS. In many institutions, the CNS is not subordinate to the manager but the manager contributes to the performance evaluation. Scheduling of work time is often a function of the unit manager. The ACNP's work time is not driven by unit needs but by case load and patient needs. A clear understanding by the manager of this unusual phenomenon is important.

In some institutions the number of nursing positions is fixed and includes the advanced practice roles. Under this formula, the manager would have to determine whether or not the unit could afford ACNPs. Because the ACNP has responsibilities within both the nursing and medical services, this arbitrary formulation is dysfunctional. Cost for the burden of providing care is logically shared between the two departments.

Quality maintenance and improvements are also within the responsibilities of the unit manager. A close working relationship with the ACNP permitting frank discussions of unit problems that include the staff nurses as well facilitates high quality. ACNPs can contribute to high-quality care because of their intimate system knowledge gained from having a nursing base, coupled with the responsibility for managing the care.

It is vital for the manager to have all APNs, whether they be direct or indirect, enjoying a productive relationship. Given a common background in nursing, the potential for deeper understanding of each others' needs and frustrations as well as strengths and weaknesses is strong. Faculty can contribute to this desired state by alerting students to the delicate balance of responsibilities that exists among all APNs and managers. Shared class content also contributes in this regard.

Clinical Nurse Specialists

At first glance it would appear that there are many areas of overlap and potential sources of tension between these two types of practitioners. Although some areas of interest such as education or patient care are identical, the spheres of influence are different. The ACNP is responsible for the patient plan of care. This could include spontaneous or planned educational sessions with other nurses. The CNS, on the other hand, may be responsible for the overall level of clinical expertise of the staff on a particular unit. The ACNP provides consultation in numerous patient situations with many of the staff. The CNS provides consultation for the entire unit by representing it on various hospitalwide committees and other forums. Both advanced practice roles support the staff nurse in the provision of care but in slightly different ways. Individual patient problems are addressed to the ACNP caring for a particular patient. Global or particular clinical problems with implications for many patients may be addressed by both.

ACNPs

Few nurses with direct care responsibility enjoy the luxury of interservice consultation with other nurses. Special relationships formed among the staff nurses on a unit are often based on schedule similarities or social friendships. Clinical Nurse Specialists network with each other at intra-hospital meetings and when consulting on the indirect aspects of their roles. Their contributions to each other's sphere of influence is invaluable. Acute Care Nurse Practitioners also have the opportunity to serve as consultants for each other, spanning different services within an institution based on individual expertise. For example, an ACNP with expertise in cardiology is a welcome colleague to one whose focus is primarily surgical patients. Likewise an ACNP with a focus of bone marrow transplantation serves as a resource when questions of malignancies arise in patients not on the oncology service. These interactions are indispensable to direct care providers who have primary responsibility for case management.

These types of collaboration are based upon mutual trust and respect. Opportunities to develop these relationships can be fostered during the educational process. Group, classroom and clinical activity support collegiality. Problem-based learning activities in the classroom also contribute to peer respect and understanding that should encompass the uncertainty of clinical decision making (Kassirer, 1995; Albanese & Mitchell, 1993).

Staff Nurses

For many nurses, advocating for patients with physicians is frustrating and anxiety provoking. First, there is a power differential between nurses and doctors. Second, timing may be off; the physician may appear on the unit when the nurse is engaged with another patient or elsewhere. The value system for the two disciplines is analogous but not identical. Nurses often intuit judgments about a patient that have no objective measurement and arc difficult to describe. These obstacles disappear in collaborative practice among staff nurses and ACNPs. Coming from the same disciplinary grounding, both ACNPs and bedside nurses create a special harmony that is otherwise absent.

Physician Assistants

Physician assistants (PAs) are a group frequently compared to ACNPs. They can be valuable allies on the care team but the differences in educational backgrounds are noteworthy. Physician assistants are educated with and by physicians. Their title bears witness to the focus of their practice: assistant to the physician. If nursing assistants could be as highly educated, trained, and motivated to assist nurses as PAs are to assist physicians, nurses would be indeed fortunate. It is erroneous to equate PAs to ACNPs. There are numerous areas of overlap, not unlike the overlap that exists between ACNPs, traditional CNSs, bedside nurses, and physicians. Physician assistants, however, remain assistants to physicians. They are not nurses and cannot fulfill nursing roles. Advancing the scientific base of nursing and helping to explicate mid-range nursing theory are obviously not on their agenda. Credible research studies are needed to uncover and measure some of the real differences among these two types of practitioners to correct any misconceptions.

BARRIERS TO PRACTICE

Several areas of difficulty have emerged with the deployment of ACNPs in the hospital setting. Students benefit by having as much knowledge as possible about the general issues pertaining to them all. Faculty and employers should familiarize students and graduates with these issues as the role of the ACNP continues to evolve.

Work Schedule

Most ACNP graduates were staff nurses before entering educational programs. The ACNP workweek and length of day is different from that in the nursing service. The feasibility of a fixed work period is compromised by the acuity of patients. If an emergency arises, the ACNP is expected to remain in place until it is resolved. This creates repercussions for ongoing coverage as the practitioner involved will eventually require time off duty. Currently there are insufficient numbers available or allocated within most systems to compensate for emergencies or planned absences like maternity leave and vacations. Much flexibility and tolerance are essential for a workable schedule with only marginal predictability. For individuals who are accustomed to greater control in their lives, this may be problematic.

Prescriptive Authority

Another issue that may be a barrier to practice involves the legal authority to order medications and therapeutic procedures and tests. Many states with statutes permitting prescriptive authority for nurses require master's degree preparation, study of additional pharmacology, and certification as advanced practitioners. Certification has just recently become available for ACNPs. This new certification will permit graduates to apply to their respective state regulatory bodies for the designation permitting them prescriptive authority.

Hospital regulatory bodies monitor clinical activities within their jurisdictions. Without prescriptive authority, the NP must have all orders co-signed by a physician. In acute or emergent situations, this places a hardship on the practitioners as well as the physicians and staff nurses.

Where there is no statutory or regulatory language for this advanced practice function, NPs may discover some difficulty in executing this segment of their clinical capabilities. They may be at greater risk for potential legal action than in areas where state law is clear. Differing statutory language among states nationwide is also problematic. Reciprocity of advanced practice is not similar to that of basic nursing licensure. If practitioners wish to relocate they may be forced to meet additional demands, such as a greater number of hours of formal study in pharmacology.

It is imperative for practitioners to understand the unique legal circumstances existing within their respective states. Likewise, faculty should prepare curricula so that graduates are permitted to gain prescriptive authority within their states as soon as possible following completion of their studies. Topics that should be addressed include: (1) practice regulation, (2) responsibilities of individual

practitioners within systems, (3) agreements with physician colleagues and/or partners, (4) use or misuse of any required protocols,
(5) malpractice liability insurance, and (6) expected changes with
health reform legislation.

Frequent Changes in Staff

The rapid change in the composition of the care team also affects
practice for the ACNP. The concept of team connotes a neatly honed
group working together. When one member is replaced, the rest of
the team feels the change.

If this change applies to a team member who manages patient
care, for example, the practitioner or a house staff member on a new
rotation, the remaining members need additional time to gauge the
treatment philosophy and judgment of the new member. This is one
of the reasons the use of NPs in providing acute care patient management is so successful; ACNPs offer more stability than was previously available.

This phenomenon also applies to the staff who are implementing
the management orders—the bedside nurses. With hospital downsizing and restructuring, regular bedside nursing staff are often aug-
mented with per-diem personnel and traveling nurses. Forced delays
occur as the management and delivery team members become
versed in each others' strengths and weaknesses. Per-diem staff may
not understand the role of the ACNP or may disagree with the
orders written by the ACNP. While these situations are rare, they
remain a source of professional frustration for the practitioner and
care team. This problem will be alleviated with increased numbers of
ACNPs holding responsibility for patient care.

ESSENTIAL ELEMENTS FOR MAINTENANCE OF THE ROLE

Despite these inherent barriers to the growth and function of the
ACNP role, the benefits are proving to far outweigh the problems.
This role is the logical next step for advanced practice nursing within
hospitals and agencies where patients are acutely ill. For the role to

be maintained in its present state and be permitted to grow, physicians, hospitals, and practitioners themselves should consider the following.

Physicians

Many physicians enthusiastically welcome this new role. They extend themselves to assist in teaching, precepting, and absorbing the new practitioner among them on the care team. A realization that someone else understands and shares the burden of directing care and that all patient problems are not straightforward serves as a foundation for a different kind of working relationship. This is one that reflects trust and collaboration. The system benefits by larger numbers of these physician colleagues.

However, not all physicians agree. Some view the ACNP role as further encroachment upon and competition with their sphere of influence. Time will permit enlightenment as they realize how valuable the ACNP contribution is to patients' well-being. Physicians need help in understanding that NPs do not wish to take over their patients but rather wish to practice to the fullest extent of their knowledge and profession.

Hospitals

In addition to the adjustments in organizational structure, credentialing, and reporting structure described above, hospitals will have to commit to the concept. A certain amount of friction is inherent in most changes, and this one is of significant magnitude. The commitment takes many forms:

- Respect—for the nursing profession in ways that have not always been historically obvious or prominent
- Protection—for the practitioner, with streamlined system policies that facilitate credentialling and suitably guard against unwarranted legal intrusion
- Nurturance—for the new role by establishing realistic expectations regarding the scope and breadth of practice responsibilities

- Compensation—for NPs that reflects the increased level of responsibilities and advanced practice skills they bring to patient care. In particular, this must be a higher salary than that paid to off-shift staff nurses.

Commitment to ACNPs is a long-term investment because the financial returns are not always immediately apparent, but the yield is high in terms of patient and nurse satisfaction. The potential is there to lower costs over time and decrease use of technology and length of stays as clinical service delivery is driven with a nursing model.

Practitioner

Three ingredients are essential to remain successful in the role of the ACNP. The first is *clinical acumen*. When one is directing the care, it is impossible and unsafe to pretend competency that does not exist. This clinical ability is predicated on a firm basis in the health sciences, particularly pathophysiology. Lengthy experience in the field also fortifies this knowledge.

Good communication skills are crucial. The ACNP is required to exchange information and ideas with a variety of caregivers as well as with the patients and families involved. The jargon of nursing is insufficient in this case. The ACNP is obliged to provide solid clinical reasoning for any ideas offered or decisions made in a logical algorithmic fashion and this is often done under stress.

Perhaps the most important element is a *deep understanding of nursing*—what it is as well as what it is not. Without this knowledge it is possible to slip away from nursing's essence and become a technician or substitute for a physician. The term "physician extender" comes to mind. There are areas of practice that do indeed overlap with physicians, but an acute care nurse practitioner is an advanced practice nurse. The more correct metaphor is an extender of nursing.

REFERENCES

Albanese, M. A., & Mitchell, S. (1993). Problem-based learning: A review of literature on its outcomes and implementation issues. *Academic Medicine, 68,* 52–81.

Benner, P. (1983). *From novice to expert.* Menlo Park, CA: Addison Wesley.

Don, M. M. (1944). Science integration in a problem-based nursing curriculum. *Research and development in problem based learning, 2,* 61–78. Australia Problem Based Learning Network.

Gunn, I. (1983). Professional territoriality and the anesthesia experience. In B. Bullough, V. Bullough, & M. C. Soukup (Eds.), Nursing issues and nursing strategies for the eighties (155–168). New York: Springer Publishing Co.

Hayes, E., & Harrell, C. (1994). On being a mentor to nurse practitioner students: The preceptor-student relationship. *Nurse Practitioner Forum, 5*(4), 220–26.

Joint Commission on Accreditation of Hospitals. (1995). *Accreditation manual for hospitals.* Chicago: Author.

Kassirer, J. P. (1995). Teaching problem-solving—how are we doing? *New England Journal of Medicine, 332*(22): 1507–1509.

Manning, D. M., Olmesdahl, P. J., Philpott, R. H., Friedman, I., & Loening, W. E. K. (1994). Towards curricular reform: Introduction of PBL concepts to faculty. *Research and Development in Problem Based Learning, 2,* 117–124. Australia Problem Based Learning Network.

Phipps, W. J., Cassmeyer, V. L., Sands, J. K., & Lehman, M. K. (1995). *Medical-surgical nursing* (5th ed). St. Louis: Mosby.

Shah, H., & Polifroni, E. C. (1992.) Precepting clinical nurse graduate students: An exploratory study. *Clinical Nurse Specialist Journal, 6*(1), 41–46.

Silver, H. K., Ford, L. C., & Day, L. R. (1968). The pediatric nurse-practitioner program: Expanding the role of the nurse to provide increased health care for children. *Journal of the American Medical Association, 204*(4), 298–302.

Trevitt, C., & Grealish, L. (1994). Learning to crawl: Development of problem based learning as a teaching strategy. *Research and Development in Problem Based Learning, 2,* 307–314. Australia Problem Based Learning Network.

Chapter **6**

AN ADMINISTRATIVE PERSPECTIVE ON THE ACUTE CARE NURSE PRACTITIONER ROLE

Kathleen M. Parrinello, PhD, RN

Hospital and health care delivery systems are being restructured throughout the United States at such a rapid pace that the only certainty in the health care system of today is that change will occur. Change is being driven by two important factors—cost and access. The inability and unwillingness of the public (individuals, employers, payers) to continue to foot the bill for rapidly rising health care costs is clearly the most pressing of these factors because access problems cannot adequately be addressed until cost is controlled.

What type of changes are occurring in health care delivery systems and how are nurses being affected? These important questions have been addressed in detail in chapter 3. However, for purposes of this discussion, it is important to emphasize several changes that have had great influence on the evolution of advanced nursing practice. First, the use of settings to describe nursing roles is becoming less relevant with the emergence of integrated delivery systems in which patients are triaged across settings to most cost effectively meet their clinical care needs. In response to this, APNs must be versatile in providing patient care in the hospital, in the ambulatory setting, in the home, and in any other location where health care services are needed. The creation of setting-based ACNP (e.g., inpatient; outpatient) roles will not position nurses to provide clinical leadership in managing continuity of care in the emerging health care delivery systems of the future.

Second, attempts to narrowly define the role, function, and clinical activities of APNs to distinguish them from other care providers will only serve to limit the evolution of the advanced nursing practice. This would be detrimental in a system in which integration and comprehensive care are required and interdisciplinary teamwork with shared responsibility for outcomes is mandatory.

In the current health care environment, APNs have the potential to take on roles of clinical leadership in the design and implementation of care delivery systems that are cost-effective and that produce the desired patient outcomes of optimal health and well-being. This chapter will be devoted to administrative issues related to the evolution of the APN role to address acute and specialty-based health care problems. It is based on the experience of the University of Rochester Medical Center, Strong Memonal Hospital, which was one of the early institutions to adopt the ACNP role. Five content areas will be addressed: Advanced practice nursing roles, organizational models for advanced practice nursing, institutional processes to support advanced practice, integration of ACNPs in the care delivery system, and compensation and funding issues.

ACNP AND CNS—MERGING OR DIFFERENTIATED ROLES?

Advanced Practice Nurses who carry the functional title of CNS have been practicing in the acute care setting since the 1960s (Elder & Bullough, 1990). The role was established to improve the quality of care delivered to acute or chronically ill patients, as well as to keep the expert, specialized nurse at the bedside. This was important because the only career advancement opportunities for nurses previously were into administrative or educational roles which required a shift in emphasis away from direct patient care. The CNS as an advanced practitioner has a primary focus on the health care system and patient care from an aggregate perspective. That is, the primary emphasis in the CNS role is to meet the needs of patients by analyzing and improving upon the systems in place for providing patient care, to provide relevant and state-of-the-art educational programs and opportunities for nurses and other health care staff, and to develop clinical policies, procedures and patient/family educational materials to assure that clinical practice is research based. The provision of direct care to individual patients and families is typically the secondary focus of the CNS role and is often provided through a consultative framework in relation to a specific, complex patient care or patient management issue. Clinical Nurse Specialists possess a specialty knowledge base in a specific area of clinical practice (e.g., critical care, musculo-skeletal, wound and skin management, etc.). To this extent, CNSs frequently are found working across clinical settings as consultants to other nurses or health care team members (Walton, Jakobowski, & Barnsteiner, 1993).

The NP role (in acute or primary care) contrasts with the CNS role in that its primary focus is on direct patient care with a secondary emphasis on delivery system issues. As depicted in Figure 6.1, both

Nurse Practitioner

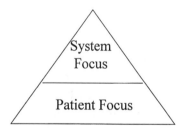

- direct patient care including physical and pyschosocial assessment, health history, diagnosis, treatment

Clinical Nurse Specialist

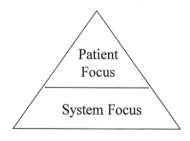

- education
- clinical research
- system improvement
- outcomes management

FIGURE 6.1   APN role objectives.

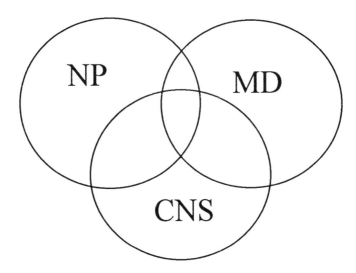

FIGURE 6.2   NP, CNS, MD role relationships.

Source: King, K., Parrinello, K., & Baggs, J. Collaboration and Collaborative Models of Practice. Philadelphia: J. B. Lippincott Co. Reprinted with permission.

types of advanced practitioners require a similar overall knowledge base. The distinction is in the emphasis placed on one aspect of the role versus the other in the clinical work setting.

Figure 6.2 presents and clarifies the complementary relationships between the NP, the CNS and the physician in the health care system. All make essential contributions to patient care. The relationship between the physician and the NP will be explored later as it relates to direct patient care. Figure 6.2 presents a model which depicts areas of overlap between the ACNP and CNS and areas of unique contribution. ACNPs increasingly are being hired by hospital organizations and other health care delivery systems to manage patients throughout specific episodes of illness. In this capacity, ACNPs work closely with physicians, nurses, and other providers to deliver direct care to patients. As advanced practitioners, ACNPs are also expected to educate others through information-sharing during patient rounds and to provide leadership in making changes in the care delivery process to improve patient outcomes. CNSs continue to be employed by hospitals and health networks in roles where they provide staff education, consultation regarding specific patient problems, and expertise in the development of clinical policies, procedures, and patient/family educational materials. As health systems adopt case management strategies to facilitate achievement of financial objectives, CNSs also are being utilized to take on the roles of case manager or outcomes management coordinator (Luquire & Houston, 1995).

With the growing imperative to provide high-quality health care at controlled costs, the challenge is to determine the most effective personnel complement to achieve the objectives of the organization. Historically, the primary types of APNs employed by hospitals were CNSs and nurse anesthetists, with NPs frequently employed by group practices or ambulatory health centers to provide outpatient services (Ray & Hardin, 1995). As the role of the ACNP develops, it is likely that some CNS positions will be reconfigured to ACNP positions, particularly if the emphasis is shifting toward more direct patient care. However, given the importance of expertise devoted to delivery system improvements, training and consultation, and systems management, the CNS will continue to play an important role in the acute care setting.

This role will include components of the special care consultant, professional educator, quality improvement coordinator, and systems manager. As organizations move away from highly centralized and functionally departmentalized structures to decentralized organizations in which clinical and programmatic decision making occurs among interdisciplinary self-managed work teams, there will be an opportunity for the CNS to apply expertise as the interdisciplinary team member, providing resource and leadership not only within the nursing department but within the organization at large.

It will be important for the nursing profession to continue to prepare nurses at the graduate level for a myriad of roles. These include indirect care roles designed to provide professional education, patient/family education, program development, outcome management, as well as graduate level practitioners who provide leadership in direct patient care. Although both CNSs and ACNPs may provide all of these services, the distinction in roles is in their primary emphasis. This will be determined largely by the way the job is configured within the health care setting. Positions emerging for advanced practice nurses that have a primary emphasis on the direct patient care responsibilities of diagnosing and treating illness as well as ordering therapeutic treatments and medications will require practitioners who take on the ACNP functional role. Positions requiring advanced practice skills that have a primary emphasis on specialty care consultation, development and implementation of professional education programs, clinical research and system analysis and improvement will go to APNs with the functional role of CNS.

This distinction in terminology regarding functional titles of APNs is not consistent in the literature on advanced practice nursing. There has been a long-standing tradition to refer to any acute care, inpatient practitioner as a CNS. Concomitantly, the term NP has long been used to reference only the primary care NP (King, Parrinello, & Baggs, in press). This terminology is problematic because it has a setting-specific connotation that is outdated in the current health care environment. As an alternative, the model presented in Figure 6.1 proposes to apply ACNP and CNS titles based on the primary emphasis of the work responsibilities and an emphasis on the complementary relationship which contributes to comprehensive care in the complex health care environment of today.

Interdisciplinary Collaboration in the APN Role

Collaboration has been described as "nurses and physicians cooperatively working together, sharing responsibility for solving problems and making decisions to formulate and carry out plans for patient care" (Baggs & Schmitt, 1988, p. 145). According to Thomas (1976) collaboration combines the activities of cooperation, or concern for the other's interests, with assertiveness, or concern for one's own interests. In the health care environment the concept of collaboration requires a mutual orientation toward the desired patient outcome and an understanding that optimal patient outcomes are achieved only when the contributions of all professionals involved in patient care are carefully coordinated. In this sense, results of collaborative practice are synergistic in that the contributions of each professional participant are optimized to a level that would not be achievable through independent practice (Weiss & Davis, 1985).

The American Nurses Association (ANA) in its document on *Nursing—A Social Policy Statement* (1980, p. 7) defines collaboration as a "true partnership, in which the power on both sides is valued by both, with recognition and acceptance of separate and combined spheres of activity and responsibility, mutual safeguarding of the legitimate interest of each party, and a commonality of tools that is recognized by both parties." Additionally, the ANA identifies interprofessional consultation and collaboration as the most appropriate mode of interaction between health care practitioners.

King, Parrinello, and Baggs (in press) propose a model for collaboration in advanced practice nursing. The authors describe two applications of collaboration that play out differently for the primary care NP and the ACNP. In the case of the primary care NP, collaboration occurs through consultation with or referral to a physician in managing patients across the continuum of care. That is, a patient has access to the services of either the primary care NP or a physician, dependent upon the patient's need at a given point in time. The NP has authority and responsibility to manage independently the care of a patient within the NP scope of practice. Collaboration comes into play for those patient needs that are outside the professional's scope of practice. In primary care, many individual patient encounters can be managed independently by the NP with referrals or consultation occurring only when patient needs require physician care. This application is based on studies that show the NP can safely and effectively manage many primary care encounters independently, in essence substituting for the need for a physician encounter (Safriet, 1992).

In contrast, the collaborative practice model in acute care is predicated on the notion that the patient's needs are such that the contributions of different types of providers are needed simultaneously to manage an episode of illness. To adequately and safely meet the patient's care needs, there can be less substitution of one provider for another. For example, the ACNP could not substitute for the surgeon who performs an operative procedure and a surgeon could not substitute for the ACNP who has responsibility for patient teaching and discharge planning (Norsen, Opladen, & Quinn, 1995).

Figure 6.3 from King, Parrinello, and Baggs (in press) depicts the difference in application of the collaborative practice model in primary versus acute care.

The circles represent patient needs or problems as well as the health care activities or functions that address the patient needs. The amount the circles overlap represents patient needs or problems that can be addressed in an equally effective manner by either type of provider. The non-overlapping part of the circles represents those patient needs or problems that are within the principal domain of one type of provider. These principal domain needs can not be addressed as well (if at all) by the other type of provider. The scope of practice of each type of provider is defined by his or her discipline and education.

Note that just because a need or activity fits into an overlapping portion of the circle, it does not mean that that need would be addressed in the same way by a different type of provider. Griffith (1984) speaks to the overlap in nurses' and physicians' functions and notes that different providers may perform the same general function but will approach it in different ways based on their unique professional perspective or experience. However, regardless of approach, for areas of overlap, each provider type should be able to produce the desired outcome.

This model presents the notion that the substitutive application appropriately describes collaborative practice in primary care whereas the complementary application better describes acute care practice. This distinction is important in understanding the continuum, along which collaborative practice arrangements are developed. The nature of the patient's care needs and the clinical requirements are key variables in understanding the degree of substitution versus complementation—not in assessing the level of collaboration. Collaborative practice can and should be developed in both applications. However, problems can arise when an application of one type of practice is misapplied to another. When this happens, the NP can be hindered from practicing to the full extent of her or his scope.

In the acute care scenario, it has been a popular notion that NPs can substitute for physician house officers (Mallison, 1993; Mundinger, 1994). Although this growing awareness throughout the hospital industry has provided the nursing profession with a window of opportunity to provide acute and specialty care in APN roles, it is essential that nursing leaders clearly articulate the complementary model of ACNP practice. That is, a portion of ACNP practice can effectively substitute for physician house staff. The full scope of

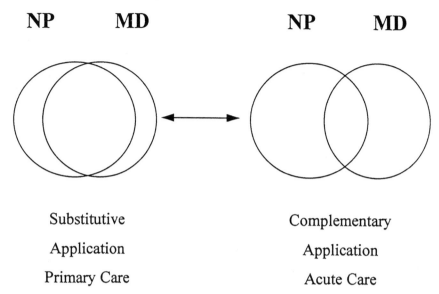

FIGURE 6.3   Application of collaboration along a continuum.
Source: Adapted from King, Parrinello, Baggs (in press). Used with permission.

ACNP practice, however, encompasses much more than a house staff substitute role because it also encompasses the practice of nursing. The unfortunate consequence of a purely substitutive model is that the full scope of the ACNP is not recognized in that the nursing functions are truncated. In addition, as a resident substitute, the APN is put in the position of being perceived as being supervised by the attending physician as opposed to being a collaborating partner.

ORGANIZATIONAL MODELS FOR ADVANCED PRACTICE NURSING IN ACUTE CARE

Institutions have adopted various organizational models to incorporate the role of nurses in advanced practice positions (Parrinello,

1995). Each model has its potential advantages and disadvantages and should be evaluated and considered in terms of its influence on a collaborative work relationship among providers, including physicians and nurses. Because the focus of this text is on the application of concepts to the ACNP functional role, organizational structures will be discussed in the context of ACNP practice.

Physician-Based Model

The first organizational model to be described is perhaps the oldest and most traditional in design. This is the physician-based model in which the ACNP joins a physician group or individual practice and establishes a working relationship with physician(s) based on the ACNP's ability to negotiate role and responsibilities. The ACNP reports administratively to a physician director. Clinical responsibilities of the ACNP typically involve the evaluation and treatment of patients referred to the specialty practice as well as the care and management of hospitalized patients including discharge planning and postdischarge follow-up care.

This model can be advantageous in that the clinical practice of the ACNP is readily interwoven with that of the medical staff. Disadvantages of the physician model include the potential tension resulting from differences in how the relationship is perceived as it relates to collaboration versus supervision. For example, the physician may perceive the MD as having ultimate authority over all aspects of patient care and all aspects of the ACNP role. Differences in understanding both the behavior required in collaborative practice and the importance of collaboration in practice may interfere with the formation of an interdependent practice in which authority and accountability for patient care management and decision making rests on competence, not upon historical medical dominance.

In this organizational structure, the substitutive application is likely to predominate because the ACNP role is directed by the physician. The areas of the ACNP's patient care management that overlap with the physician's may be emphasized over other role components, especially if physician resources are stretched thin. In addition, this organizational model could result in isolation of the ACNP from nursing colleagues if the ACNP role is configured as part of the physician group practice. This in turn could result in a loss of credibility of the ACNP among nursing staff in the clinical setting as nurses come to view the ACNP as a physician extender instead of an advanced practice nurse with expertise in the nursing care needs of patients.

Another concern identified with this type of organizational model is the degree to which the work of the ACNP can be directed by the physician toward office support activities such as coordinating referrals, directing patients, and processing forms and letters (Phillips, Spaulding, & O'Neal, 1995). The result would be an underutilization of the ACNP for complex, skilled, direct patient care activities, creating role dissatisfaction and cost inefficiencies.

Nursing Model

A second type of organizational model for ACNP practice is the nursing model in which the ACNP reports to a nursing director and is assigned to work with physicians to address clinical care issues (Parrinello, 1995). This model represents the traditional CNS model and can be useful for ACNP practice in specialized units, such as emergency departments or critical care units; advantages include the development of a strong and clear identification with nursing and nursing issues which enhances the credibility of the ACNP among nursing staff. In addition, this model may offer an increased opportunity to maintain a secondary focus on indirect advanced practice nursing activities such as consultation, clinical teaching, and systems improvement as well as the primary focus on direct patient care.

Disadvantages of the nursing model include the potential for decreased collaboration with physicians if the ACNP is perceived to be functioning separately from the physician instead of being part of the patient care team. Phillips, Spaulding, and O'Neal (1995) describe the challenge associated with creating a management structure for APNs that is consistent with the concept of physician and nurse collaboration held by the medical leadership of the organization. Disadvantages of this model can be minimized by assuring that the ACNP's indirect care responsibilities are complementary to and carefully balanced with direct care clinical responsibilities. In addition, a clearly defined collaborative practice agreement developed between the ACNP and the physician partner(s) is an important component that can clarify accountabilities and responsibilities within the joint practice relationship.

Another disadvantage of this model may stem from cost-accounting issues if ACNP positions are rolled into the large nursing personnel budget of the institution. In this case, accurate cost accounting by clinical program may be difficult to achieve. It is important in this environment of case-based reimbursement that the contributions of ACNPs to effective patient-care management, such as decreasing lengths of hospital stay, avoiding unnecessary hospital admission, and managing variances in the care delivery process and patients' responses to care, are carefully documented.

Collaborative Practice Model

The third organizational model that is emerging is the joint-practice model of collaborative practice (Richmond & Keane, 1992; Walton, Jakobowski, & Barnsteiner, 1993; Parrinello, 1995). In this model, the physician and the ACNP as a team provide care to patients and share authority and accountability for providing that care within their respective scopes of practice. A cohesive physician-nurse clinical care delivery model is cultivated, and the communication structure between physicians and ACNPs is formalized. Reporting relationships are developed within a matrix management model in which the ACNP is responsible to a physician director for many clinical care issues and to a nursing director for issues relating to professional practice, program development, and system improvement. Advantages of this model reflect the advantages of both the physician- and the nursing-based models because, by design, it is an attempt to capture the best of both approaches. The concept of interdependency is emphasized, and the goal is to achieve coordination of care and integration of services within a health care delivery system.

Disadvantages of the joint-practice model include the complexity that is associated with matrix organizational models and the potential for the practitioner to get caught between two professional viewpoints regarding the priorities of the role. In the complex health care environment of today, however, it is essential that clinical leaders create organizational models that optimize productivity and practitioner development and reflect the professional interdependence required to deliver high-quality and cost-effective health care services.

The ACNP role at the University of Rochester Medical Center, Strong Memorial Hospital (URMCSMH), was developed in 1979 with the appointment of an ACNP to the cardiac surgery service (Davitt & Jensen, 1981). This advanced practice role has evolved into a nationally recognized prototype for advanced nursing practice in the acute care setting (Ackerman, Norsen, Martin, Wiedrich, & Kitzman, 1995). At Strong Memorial, a joint-practice model best describes the organizational structure for advanced nursing practice.

The role of the ACNP, in this model, encompasses comprehensive direct patient care, systems support, scholarly practice, and profes-

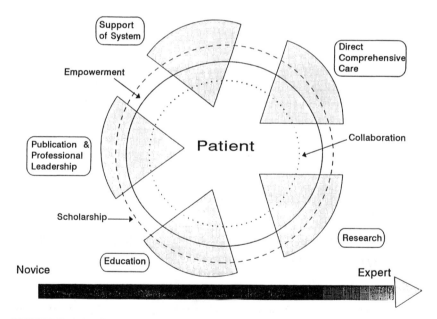

FIGURE 6.4   Strong Model of Advanced Practice.

Source: © University of Rochester, Strong Memorial Hospital. Reprinted with permission.

sional leadership (Figure 6.4). The direct care responsibilities of the ACNP at Strong Memorial include recording patient health histories and performing complete physical exams and psychosocial assessments, ordering and performing diagnostic testing and screening, diagnosing illness, prescribing both pharmacologic and other treatments for patients, and providing health maintenance and promotion interventions such as patient and family education and counseling. Systems support involves activities that promote innovative patient care practices and facilitate the optimal progression of patients through the health care system. Quality improvement activities are an important component of the domain of systems support. Scholarly practice includes the use of research findings to continuously improve patient care and the generation of new knowledge through use of scientific methods. Responsibility for contributing to the education of future practitioners is inherent in the concept of scholarship and is an important component of the model. Professional leadership requires the dissemination of knowledge generated within an area of expertise beyond the confines of the individual practitioner's clinical practice setting. Required behaviors include publication in the professional literature and presentation of information and findings to professional groups.

Providing unity to this model are the three conceptual strands of collaboration, empowerment and scholarship. In addition, a continuum of expertise lies at the base of the model and is premised on Benner's (1984) work. The continuum, from novice to expert, represents the degree of proficiency within the domains of practice and the degree of mastery in the application of the conceptual strands in all aspects of the role.

INSTITUTIONAL PROCESSES TO SUPPORT ACNP ROLE DEVELOPMENT

Institutions can and should create supportive environments that facilitate and enhance collaborative practice among physicians, ACNPs, and other health team members. In addition to organizational structure, other important components of a supportive environment include effective administrative processes that establish and recognize appropriate scope of practice and that guide clinical privileging and performance review of ACNPs.

As mentioned earlier, ACNPs have graduate degrees in clinical nursing and are recognized through certification or licensure to practice in an expanded capacity which includes diagnosis and treatment of health conditions. The role of the ACNP encompasses comprehensive, direct patient care reflecting expert, specialty-based practice and conforming to professional practice standards. Professional organizations, such as the American Nurses Association, have led the way in articulating standards to guide the clinical practice of nursing and nursing administration. With the evolution of the ACNP role, an ANA task force was convened in 1993 to establish a "Scope of Acute Care Advanced Nursing Practice and Standards of Acute Care Advanced Nursing Practice." The standards were completed and published in 1995. They reflect the current practice of ACNPs that has emerged in a number of settings across the country; they clarify the scope of practice for ACNPs and provide a framework for the development of future ACNP roles.

Scope of Practice and Practice Standards:
One Organization's Perspective

Table 6.1 depicts a condensed version of the Scope of Practice and Professional Practice Standards developed by the ACNPs and nursing leadership at Strong Memorial Hospital. The Scope of Practice is a statement of expectations regarding practice responsibilities and outlines in very broad terms those elements that define advanced nursing practice. A comprehensive understanding of the Scope of practice is essential for all members on the health care team, since the legal parameters for a collaborative practice agreement require practicing within one's professional scope. While most elements of the Scope of Practice are practitioner specific, there are areas of overlap between medical practice and advanced nursing practice (refer to Figure 6.3) that should be negotiated between the physician and the ACNP to eliminate duplication and redundancy in services provided to patients cared for by a team (Norsen, Opladen, & Quinn, 1995).

TABLE 6.1 University of Rochester / Strong Memorial Hospital Surgical Nursing Practice Acute Care Nurse Practitioner Professional Practice Standards

Scope of Practice

The Acute Care Nurse Practitioner (ACNP) is an advanced practice nurse who functions in an expanded nursing role in a Collaborative Practice Model. The ACNP has completed graduate education in nursing science and demonstrates a comprehensive knowledge base in a specialty practice area exhibiting a high level of clinical competence in caring for acutely ill patients. The ACNP provides patient care utilizing advanced assessment skills and a sound knowledge of clinical therapeutics. The ACNP provides indirect patient care services to support patient care, promote professional education and advance knowledge through research and scholarly activities. All duties and responsibilities of the ACNP conform to professional practice standards, hospital guidelines, and are in accordance with a written practice agreement with a physician member of the Medical Staff at the University of Rochester, Strong Memorial Hospital.

	Standard	Rationale
I.	Entry into Acute Care	The ACNP facilitates entry of the patient into the acute care system at the first contact.	Effective entry into the acute care system ensures the identification and management of the presenting concern and establishes a mechanism for anticipating and dealing with future patient care needs, which may arise during the episode of acute care.
II.	Comprehensive Care	The ACNP provides direct care that is comprehensive, continuous, coordinated, and accessible throughout hospitalization and after discharge.	Comprehensive care includes timely assessment, intervention, and promotes quality outcomes for the patient while decreasing the cost of health care.

		The ACNP provides indirect care that supports care delivery systems, promotes education, and advances scholarly practice.	
III.	Interdisciplinary Practice	The ACNP collaborates with other health care providers in caring for patients within a given specialty population.	Interdisciplinary practice utilizes the expertise of all health care professionals to ensure delivery of quality care.
IV.	Continuing Competence	The ACNP assumes responsibility for maintaining competence in a specialty area.	Theory and knowledge of health care and disease management increases at a rapid rate. Because technology advances continuously, the skills necessary to practice safely and effectively must be reviewed and updated regularly.
V.	Quality Assessment and Improvement	The ACNP provides leadership in quality assessment and quality improvement activities in the acute care setting.	Participation in quality improvement activities promotes excellence in the delivery of patient care in the acute care setting.
VI.	Research/Scholarly Practice	The ACNP supports scholarly practice by integrating research into practice, by providing leadership in a specialty area, and by educating students.	Scholarly practice enhances professional growth and quality patient outcomes.

Source: University of Rochester, Strong Memorial Hospital. Reproduced with permission.

Standards of practice are an operationalism of the Scope of Practice and are clear and specific statements outlining activities or behaviors that constitute daily practice. At Strong Memorial, the standards developed for the ACNP provide a delineation of the domains identified above. The condensed version of the six standards of practice developed for the surgical ACNP group also are contained in Table 6.1. The standards of practice provide the framework for outcome measurement and individual performance review of the ACNP. Performance criteria for all professional nurses include professional practice requirements, care delivery requirements, and requirements for clinical coordination such as case management activities, program development, and systems improvement. Table 6.2 presents the major performance criteria categories and examples of required behaviors. A system for professional advancement of nurses (SPAN) has been developed at Strong Memorial and the role requirements for ACNPs have been developed within this professional practice model (Clements & Parrinello, in press). Given the breadth and depth of these job requirements, the ACNP role has been placed at the highest level in the clinical track of the SPAN.

The expanded clinical role of ACNPs has caused many organizations to develop internal systems of credential review for ACNPs and other advanced practitioners. These systems often mirror the review procedure applied to physicians requesting practice privileges within an organization (Quigley, Hixon, & Jangen, 1991; Smith, 1991). Credential review is important as it provides organizations with a mechanism to assure that only practitioners with the appropriate level of expertise and skill are permitted to practice under the auspices of the organization. As nurses in increasing numbers are undergoing this kind of review, it is essential for organizations to establish multidisciplinary review teams to review credentials and evaluate appropriateness of appointment.

At Strong Memorial, an interdisciplinary review procedure has been established for appointment of nurses with expanded practice privileges consistent with the scope of practice for APNs. The review procedure, described in detail by Smith (1991), incorporates several key steps and processes.

Upon appointment to the institution, all APNs (NP, CNM, CRNA, CNS) are required to submit a formal request for practice

TABLE 6.2 University of Rochester / Strong Memorial Hospital Surgical Nursing Practice Performance Criteria for Acute Care Nurse Practitioners

			Performance Criteria
PROFESSIONAL PRACTICE	Professional involvement in group activity	A.	Influences the direction and outcome of group activities at the unit/service level.
		B.	Actively participates in professional organizations.
	Scholarly activities	A.	Facilitates clinical research through collaboration with others in investigations, analysis of practice problems to generate researchable questions, and enabling access to clients and data.
		B.	Assists others in applying scientific knowledge to nursing practice and clinical decision making.
		C.	Disseminates nursing knowledge through presentation or publication at the local/regional level.
	Role Development	A.	Maintains a current knowledge base in area of specialization.
		B.	Develops and implements plan for professional growth and development.
	Professional Image/ Interpersonal Skills	A.	Enhances care delivery by serving as a mentor for others.
		B.	Promotes nursing and quality patient care when interacting with other professionals, patients/families, and the public.
		C.	Represents nursing positively in recruitment and retention activities.

continued

TABLE 6.2 *Continued*

		Performance Criteria
CARE DELIVERY	Direct/Indirect Care	A. Assesses the quality and effectiveness of the nursing care delivery system in assigned specialty area.
		B. Delivers direct care and coordinates interdisciplinary plan of care for patients requiring the expertise of an advanced practitioner.
		C. Provides leadership in the development, implementation, and evaluation of standards of practice, policies, and procedures.
		D. Facilitates the process of ethical decision making in clinical practice.
	Consultation	Serves as a consultant in improving patient care and nursing practice based on expertise in area of specialization.
CLINICAL COORDINATION	Education	A. Applies teaching/learning theory to patient, family, community, and professional education as a means to influence patient outcomes.
		B. Identifies learning needs of various populations and contributes to the development of educational programs/resources.

	C.	Serves as a formal educator and clinical preceptor for students, staff, and/or others.
	D.	Participates in School of Nursing activities as negotiated.
Quality Improvement/ Critical Analysis	A.	Identifies system-specific problems requiring evaluation or change.
	B.	Participates in strategic planning for the practice area/ service.
	C.	Provides direction for and participates in unit/service quality improvement programs.
	D.	Evaluates impact of changes in clinical practice and formulates recommendations regarding appropriateness and cost-effectiveness.
Program Development		Actively participates in the development, implementation, and evaluation of practice-related programs in collaboration with nursing leadership.

Source: University of Rochester, Strong Memorial Hospital. Reproduced with permission.

privileges encompassing all direct patient care services that they will provide. Advanced practice nurses not employed by the institution but employed by a group practice admitting patients to Strong Memorial or another community health care agency involved with patient care at Strong must also formally request practice privileges before gaining access to patients. This request is submitted to the nursing clinical chief along with letters of recommendation, the practitioner's curriculum vitae, proof of licensure as an RN, and documentation of advanced practice certification. The Scope of Practice statement (see Table 6.1) and a practice-specific procedure/skills list are also submitted. In New York State, NPs are certified by the state upon meeting given educational requirements and submitting a written practice agreement with a licensed physician that describes broadly defined clinical protocols upon which the collaborative practice is based. A copy of this written practice agreement is required for the credentials review process.

Upon submission of all required materials, the clinical nursing chief and the medical chief of the appropriate clinical service (e.g., surgery, pediatrics, etc.) review all documentation and recommend approval of practice privileges. The professional practice committee of the nursing organization also reviews and endorses the practice privilege request. On a quarterly basis, the institutional clinical leadership committee reviews all endorsed applicants and formally grants practice privileges. Privileges are reviewed one year following the initial appointment and every two years thereafter.

An important component of the ongoing review process is the annual performance evaluation that is coordinated by the nursing clinical chief/designee and incorporates quality assessment data as well as feedback from physicians and nurses practicing with the ACNP. For the ACNP employed by Strong Memorial, the performance review process includes a detailed self-assessment addressing each of the advanced practice performance criteria listed in Table 6.2. This self-assessment is abbreviated for ACNPs employed by another agency because many of the performance criteria address contributions to the ongoing growth and development of the organization. Both groups of ACNPs, however, are required to participate in departmental quality assessments where patient care is reviewed and adherence to the standards of practice is measured. Finally, ACNPs are required to submit peer reviews by a collaborating physician and nurse as an important component of the annual performance review process.

Integration of ACNPs in Acute Care Delivery Systems

The integration of ACNPs into the organization's care delivery system should be deliberately and carefully executed before the role of the ACNP is actually implemented. Failure to do this may result in redundancy of effort, role confusion, and dissatisfaction on the part of the ACNP. In addition, resentment or frustration may emerge among other members of the health care team if roles are not carefully introduced. In this continually changing environment, ACNP role descriptions should be developed broadly with less emphasis on specific tasks or procedures to be performed than on the purpose of the role in contributing to optimal patient care outcomes.

Ideally, the organization that incorporates the ACNP into the care delivery system has made a commitment to patient-centered care as an organizing principle for care delivery and collaborative practice as the organizing principle for professional behavior. In the context of patient-centered care, the ongoing assessment and validation of patient/family care needs is the focus of goal setting and decision making regarding care delivery. The creation of interdisciplinary health care teams to manage care for specific patient populations is an essential structural element in the effective operationalization of collaborative practice.

Depending on the typical needs of the patient population, the collaborative team may include any number of health care professionals including physicians, ACNPs, RNs, physical therapists, social workers, occupational therapists, pharmacists, dieticians and other specialty-care providers. Consistency in team membership is important for the development of cohesive and effective interdisciplinary teams in which participants gain familiarity in working with each other and become committed as individuals to the group effort required of the team. To achieve consistency in team membership, organizational barriers resulting from highly centralized and departmentalized organizational structures must be eliminated. This is necessary to support work teams that comprise a cross-section of professionals whose contributions must be highly coordinated to organize and manage patient care across the health care continuum.

The format, policies, and procedures relating to documentation of patient care support a collaborative team approach to patient care. A medical record in which clinical documentation from all team members is integrated is an important component of interdisciplinary practice. Patient clinical data should be collected in a systematic and ongoing fashion and include the assessments of all appropriate health team members. Forms or systems used in documentation should consolidate medical and nursing information as much as possible to improve efficiency, reduce redundancy, and facilitate comprehensive assessment and relevant care planning. Institutional policies for order writing, including diagnostic and laboratory testing, therapeutic interventions, medications and consult requests, must be developed to enable the ACNP to perform in the advanced practice role consistent with the established scope of practice.

Compensation Issues for the ACNP

Currently, there is no direct reimbursement mechanism for ACNPs who provide care during the hospital episode. ACNPs, unlike nurse anesthetists, nurse midwives, and physicians, cannot bill patients or payers a professional fee for care they provide as part of a hospital admission. Therefore, existing hospital inpatient reimbursement systems must cover the services provided by ACNPs. In the current case-based payment system, this may be perceived as a barrier to expanding ACNP practice in the hospital setting because the ACNP is another expense against a fixed hospital revenue stream. To the extent the ACNP is able to reduce other expenses associated with hospitalization, such as decreasing length of stay and/or reducing use of ancillary or high-cost pharmaceutical therapy, the added salary expense becomes a financially sound investment.

In addition, most health care financing reform initiatives, in both the public and private sector, are based on capitated contracting as the payment mechanism of the future. Under capitation, patient care may no longer be reimbursed separately for both the hospital and provider components of service. Instead, payment will occur based on the enrollment of persons in the plan and the health care system must manage the health care needs of those enrolled over a continuum of care geared toward cost-effective utilization, not volume of services provided (Cerne, 1994). Revenue from enrolled persons typically is divided between the hospital, professional providers, and any other component of the system, such as home health care. Providers are paid a salary and share in the benefits and the risks of the plan. In this environment, the ACNP has tremendous potential as a health care professional who is affordable and versatile, bridging the gap between medicine and nursing and promoting continuity in care delivery across settings.

As discussed earlier, in the hospital setting ACNPs have been employed to perform many of the services for which resident physicians typically have been responsible. It is important to emphasize, however, that this is not solely a substitutive role because ACNPs also provide important services (continuity and clinical coordination) that have not been part of the resident physicians' responsibilities. In fact, in the acute care setting, ACNPs can complement attending physician services by integrating the nursing component of care with the medical plan of care to achieve a high level of coordination in care delivery. In this type of model, use of ACNPs can be an effective way to control rising costs associated with physician payments because physician specialists working in partnership with ACNPs are able to increase their caseloads without additional, more costly physician specialist partners.

It has been argued that ACNPs, when viewed as physician extenders replacing or substituting for resident physicians in tertiary care, are more costly than the exclusive use of residents. This is because residents typically work longer hours than ACNPs and their stipends are less than ACNP salaries. Whereas lower resident salaries and longer work hours make residents a less costly option when compared to an ACNP in a given year of residency, the costs of health care, over the long run, are driven upward due to the oversupply of specialists produced by an overgrowth of residency training programs. Currently, Medicare funds 40–50% of the nation's 7189 residency programs at 896 sponsoring institutions and this expense is heavily weighted toward specialization and subspecialization. Costs due to graduate medical education (GME) have risen significantly since 1965 and recent proposals to reform GME funding are aimed at reducing the expense associated with specialty residency training (Johnson, 1994).

At present ACNPs typically are salaried by the hospital or other employing agency. At Strong Memorial, a competitive salary scale has been developed for ACNPs that recognizes years of experience in nursing and years of experience as an NP. Because the ACNPs enter into a joint-practice arrangement with faculty physicians and contribute directly to the private practice revenue stream associated with physician professional practice fees, contributing funds are often negotiated from the physician practice groups to support the ACNP's salary. Given current payment systems which reimburse hospitals and providers separately, it is important for hospital and nursing administrators to carefully monitor the ACNP work effort and differentiate the ACNP care that is part of the hospital component from the ACNP care that substitutes for the provider component. Phillips, Spaulding, & O'Neal (1995) describe a system to account for the work effort of APNs at the University of Massachusetts Medical Center to determine appropriate funding sources. It is recommended that the hospital absorb the cost of ACNP care that contributes to the hospital payment component and negotiate ACNP salary support for care that is reimbursed in the provider fee component. In a capitated payment system, this distinction may be important from a productivity monitoring perspective but has little financial implication as the payment mechanism is based on enrollment in the plan, not on the type or place of service.

CONCLUSION

Both the pressures of an increasingly strained and costly health care system as well as a reorientation to a patient-centered environment have caused nursing and health care leaders to embrace the concept of an APN whose clinical practice encompasses components of both medical and nursing care. Continued growth and expansion of the ACNP role can be expected to the extent that the four following role dimensions are encouraged and supported.

First, the role must focus on integration and coordination of medical, nursing and ancillary care. Continuity is key in the complex health care environment of today. Effective referral patterns must be cultivated and information shared so that patients and families experience the seamless care they want and need and so that redundancy in resource utilization is minimized. Second, the ACNP must make a commitment to ongoing education and training. Organizations must recognize and support this need by providing the resources and programs necessary to facilitate continued competence in a variety of assessment, diagnostic, and treatment modalities as well as in retooling for new skills introduced as a result of new knowledge and technology. Third, there must be a focus on the health care needs of the population served and continual improvement of the systems within which health care is provided so that costs are controlled and access enhanced. ACNPs must draw upon skills in community assessment and system improvement to assure that affordable services are designed and delivered to meet the needs of the community. Finally, the ACNP must continuously experiment with new structures and processes of care delivery focusing on the relationship between resources consumed and outcomes achieved. Outcomes of care need to be clearly defined and monitored, along with the resources consumed to achieve those outcomes.

The development of the ACNP role is a response to the changing health care environment that is proactive and innovative. Nurse executives and health care administrators must carefully examine and support the continuous evolution of these roles in an effort to assure that patients receive a high quality of care from professionals who are most qualified and capable of providing care and accepting accountability for clinical outcomes.

REFERENCES

Ackerman, M., Norsen, L., Martin, B., Wiedrich, J., & Kitzman, H. (unpublished manuscript). *The Strong Memorial Model of Advanced Practice.*

American Nurses Association. (1980). *Nursing: A social policy statement.* Kansas City, MO: Author.

American Nurses Association. (1993). *Nursing facts, advanced practice nursing: A new age in health care.* Washington, D.C.: American Nurses Association.

Baggs, J. G., & Schmitt, M. H. (1988). Collaboration between nurses and physicians. *Image: Journal of Nursing Scholarship, 20*, 145–149.

Benner, P. (1984). *From novice to expert: Excellence and power in clinical nursing practice.* Menlo Park, CA: Addison-Wesley Publishing Co.

Cerne, F. (1994). Shaping up for capitation. *Hospitals and Health Networks, 68*(7), 28–30.

Clements, J., & Parrinello, K. (in press). Career advancement for the nurse in advanced practice. *Nursing Management.*

Consensus Conference on Preparing Nurses for Advanced Practice in Acute Care. (1993). Standards for educational programs: Preparing students as acute care nurse practitioners. *AACN Clinical Issues, 4*(4), 593–598.

Davitt, P., & Jensen, L. (1981). The role of the acute care nurse practitioner in cardiac surgery. *Nursing Administration Quarterly, 6*(1), 16–19.

Elder, R. G., & Bullough, B. (1990). Nurse practitioners and clinical nurse specialists: Are the roles merging? *Clinical Nurse Specialist, 4*(2), 78–84.

Griffith, H. (1984). Nursing practice: Substitute or complement according to economic theory. *Nursing Economic, 2*, 105–112.

Johnson, S. (1994). GME financing: A well-kept secret. *Nursing Management, 25*(4), 43–46.

King, K., Parrinello, K., & Baggs, J. (in press). Collaboration and collaborative models of practice. In J. Hickey, R. Ouimette, & S. Venegoni, *Nurse Practitioners: Moving into the 21st Century.* Philadelphia, PA: J.B. Lippincott Co.

Luquire, R., & Houston, S. (1995). *Outcomes management and research at St. Luke's Episcopal Hospital, Houston, Texas.* Presented at the Premier Health Alliance Nurse Executive Meeting, Savanah, GA, February 8–10.

Mallison, M. (1993). Nurses as house staff. *American Journal of Nursing, 93*(3), 7.

Mundinger, M.O. (1994). Advanced practice nursing—Good medicine for physicians? *New England Journal of Medicine, 330*, 211–214.

Norsen, L., Opladen, J., & Quinn, J. (1995). Practice model: Collaborative practice. *Critical Care Nursing Clinics of North America, 7*(1), 43–52.

Parrinello, K. (1995). Advanced practice nursing: An administrative perspective. *Critical Care Nursing Clinics of North America, 7*(1), 1–8.

Phillips, M., Spaulding, R., & O'Neal, L. (1995). Determining appropriate funding for advanced practice nurses. *Nursing Economic$, 13*, 12–17.

Quigley, P., Hixon, A., & Jangen, S. (1991). Promoting autonomy and professional practice: A program of clinical privileging. *Journal of Nursing Quality Assurance, 5*(3), 27–32.

Ray, G., & Hardin, S. (1995) Advanced practice nursing: Playing a vital role. *Nursing Management, 26*(2), 45–47.

Richmond, T., & Keane, A. (1992). The nurse practitioner in tertiary care. *Journal of Nursing Administration, 22*(11), 11–12.

Safriet, B. J. (1992). Health care dollars and regulatory sense: The role of advanced practice nursing. *Yale Journal on Regulation, 9,* 419–488.

Smith, T. (1991). A structured process to credential nurses with advanced practice skills. *Journal of Nursing Quality Assurance, 5*(3), 40–51.

Thomas, K. (1976). Conflict and conflict management. In M.D. Dunnette (Ed.), *Handbook of industrial and organizational psychology* (pp. 889–935). Chicago: Rand McNally College Publishing Company.

Walton, M., Jakobowski, D., & Barnsteiner, J. (1993). A collaborative practice model for the clinical nurse specialist. *Journal of Nursing Administration, 23*(2), 55–59.

Weiss, S. J., & Davis, H. P. (1985). Validity and reliability of the collaborative practice scale. *Nursing Research, 34,* 299–305.

Chapter 7

ACTUALIZATION OF THE ACNP ROLE: THE EXPERIENCE OF UNIVERSITY HOSPITALS OF CLEVELAND

Anne Gedwill, ND, MSN, RN
Sharon Mack, MSN, RN
Diane Mlakar, MSN, RN
Rachel K. Vanek, MSN, RN

University Hospitals of Cleveland (UHC) is a tertiary-care hospital with over 900 beds located on the eastern edge of Cleveland, Ohio. It comprises four specialty hospitals geographically linked under the umbrella of University Hospitals of Cleveland. The full range of adult medical and surgical, pediatric, obstetrical, and psychiatric services is offered. It is affiliated with the nursing, medical, and dental schools of Case Western Reserve University (CWRU).

Advanced practice nursing roles have been in existence at University Hospitals of Cleveland for a number of years. Advanced practice nurses (APNs) have been used in a variety of areas, including Womens' Health, Hepatology, Psychiatry, Anesthesia, Pediatrics and Family Practice. The adult medical and surgical areas have primarily used clinical nurse specialists (CNSs) while the neonatal and pediatric outpatient divisions have employed nurse practitioners (NPs). The role of the Acute Care Nurse Practitioner (ACNP) represents a new role for APNs on the inpatient adult medical and surgical divisions.

The impetus for the ACNP role arose from a myriad of changes in the health care environment (Richmond & Keane, 1992). These changes include impressive advances in medical diagnostics and therapeutics, changes in postgraduate medical education, reduction in financial support for house officer training, increased autonomy in nursing practice, and the high cost of health care delivery in teaching hospitals. All of these factors have lead to the exploration of alternatives for providing comprehensive patient care (Landefeld, Rosenthal, & Brennan, 1992). This exploration has prompted the development of the ACNP role. The purpose of this chapter is to describe how the ACNP role has developed at one hospital, University Hospitals of Cleveland. Similarities and differences in expectations, responsibilities, and barriers to practice will be discussed as illustrative of issues and challenges inherent in this new role.

PRACTICE SITES

At University Hospitals of Cleveland the four areas selected to receive the first class of ACNPs were neuroscience, oncology, medical intensive care, and adult internal medicine. Only the adult internal medicine service, as part of a pilot research project, had previously functioned with a nurse practitioner on staff.

Neuroscience

The function of the ACNP on the neuroscience division is twofold: to manage patients with a variety of neurological diseases and to implement a case management model of care. This 30-bed patient unit consists of neurological, neurosurgical and orthopedic spinal surgery patients. The neurology ward service consists of three residents and an attending neurologist, all of whom rotate monthly. The neurological team may consist of first-year neurology residents or may include rotating first-year medicine or psychiatric residents. It is the ACNP who maintains consistency for patients despite this rotation of physicians.

Within the specialty of neuroscience nursing, the ACNP's caseload varies to include management of patients with seizures, strokes, or neurodegenerative diseases. Due to the debilitating nature of stroke and the lack of aggressive interventional methods of treatment, the problems presented by these patients tend to be less appealing for residents, eager to learn new techniques of management. The ACNP has a primary focus of case-managing patients with a diagnosis of stroke by promoting the multidisciplinary care involved in this population on the neuroscience division or neuroscience intensive care unit.

Oncology

The inpatient oncology division contains two distinct subsets. The bone marrow transplant service cares for patients with "liquid" tumors such as leukemia, and any patient undergoing a bone marrow transplant. The general oncology service cares for patients with solid tumors and hematologic disorders. Although the nursing staff cares for patients of both services, the ACNP works only with patients on the general oncology service. The ACNP functions as a member of a large medical team which includes physician assistants, interns, a senior resident, an oncology fellow, and an attending physician. With the exception of the ACNP and the physician assistants, all members of the team change monthly.

The patient population consists of patients with a wide range of problems related to cancer, including the need for chemotherapy and pain management, infection, thrombotic complications, or other oncologic complications requiring emergent interventions such as spinal cord compression. In addition to oncology patients, the service admits patients with hematologic diseases, including hemophilia and sickle cell disease. Many of the patients become well known to the permanent team members and nursing staff because they are rehospitalized a number of times over the course of their illnesses.

Critical Care

The ACNP in the Medical Intensive Care Unit (MICU) is part of a multidisciplinary team caring for patients who require the intensive care setting for the management of their illnesses. The team consists of the attending physician, a pulmonary/critical care fellow, three residents, and the ACNP. The ACNP is the only member who does not rotate monthly. A core group of five attending physicians who work in the MICU provide stability and consistency among the attending physicians. Patients are admitted under the care of the MICU attending physician who directs their care while in the unit. Although the referring attending physicians make rounds and recommendations daily, it is the critical care team who manage ongoing patient care issues.

Patients are admitted to the unit with a wide variety of clinical conditions. As part of a tertiary-care center, the MICU offers specialty critical care to patients with multisystem failures which may be of an infectious, hematologic, neurologic, cardiac, pulmonary, endocrine, renal, or gastroenterologic etiology.

Adult Medicine

The adult internal medicine ACNP practices on a general internal medicine unit with a health care delivery model known as the Collaborative Clinical Service (CCS). This type of care delivery model originated from efforts exploring alternative methods of providing health care in teaching hospitals. The CCS represents a creative system in which nursing and physician work is integrated for the delivery of care and clinical decision making. An integral part of this service is a grant-funded, prospective randomized clinical trial examining patient outcomes, cost-effectiveness, and overall satisfaction of patients and health care providers with the use of ACNPs in place of house officers. The project, discussed in more detail later in this chapter, resulted from joint efforts from the Departments of Medicine and Nursing and its affiliate, Case Western Reserve University. The CCS is a 20-bed division which admits both private and staff patients, general medicine patients, and patients 18 years of age or older with cystic fibrosis. Medical residents are not utilized and patient care is managed by the division nursing staff, NPs, and the patient's private physician or, in the case of staff patients, the unit's medical director.

ROLE RESPONSIBILITIES

Although the areas in which ACNPs work are different in many respects, there are a number of common responsibilities. These include fundamental responsibilities of patient management, acting as a member of the nursing leadership group, participating in professional development activities, and serving as a teacher and mentor.

Common Components

Patient Management

Over the past 25 years, the place for NPs in the health care system has evolved despite confusion and blurring of the distinction of their role from that of medical professionals, as well as a resistance from nursing professionals regarding the advanced scope of practice. Integration of this role into the acute care setting requires a clear vision and precise articulation of the commonalities in the responsibilities regardless of clinical focus. Despite the expansion of many dimensions of care offered by advanced practitioners, one element remains central—the patient as central focus in the delivery of services. Patient management, the core of the ACNP role, has similarities that extend across specializations.

The spectrum of services begins with the ACNP's assessment of complex acutely ill patients. The process of admitting the patient to the acute care facility includes performing the initial history and physical examination, communicating with the referring physician, determining what the patient's goals are for the hospitalization, plan-

ning and performing diagnostic procedures, and developing a therapeutic plan. The plan is arrived at after collaboration with appropriate members of the team and is then communicated to everyone
involved with the patient's care through documentation in the
patient's medical record. Documentation includes the writing of
orders as well as patient notes. Because of the lack of prescriptive
authority in this state, orders are completed by the ACNP but must
be co-signed by a resident or attending physician.

Utilizing general and specialized knowledge bases, the ACNP
offers skill in diagnosis, development of therapeutic treatment re-
gimes, as well as risk-prevention measures. Following daily rounds
with a physician team, patients are managed interdependently by the
ACNP who develops his or her own caseload and manages the
patient throughout the hospital stay. Throughout the hospitalization,
the patient's primary care physician is contacted by the NP for care
recommendations, to provide patient status updates, and to discuss
follow-up plans. The ACNP initiates consultation and referrals with
other physicians, nurses, and health care professionals appropriate
for the patient's needs.

Diagnostic and therapeutic procedures required in the acutely or
critically ill patient are completed by the ACNP. Commonly performed skills in each of the ACNP practices include arterial blood
gases, phlebotomy, insertion of feeding tubes, and interpretation of
radiographic studies. In some areas the ACNPs perform other advanced procedures appropriate for their area of practice. In neuroscience, lumbar punctures (LPs) are performed by ACNP. She
independently completes this procedure on her own patients or may
use the opportunity as a teaching experience for the medical students
and rotating medical/psychiatry residents whose patients require
an LP. In the intensive care unit the ACNP is privileged to insert arterial lines, remove pulmonary artery catheters, perform para-
centesis, thoracentesis, and lumbar punctures. Specialized skills such
as these are learned through didactic instruction and demonstration.
Privileging is obtained through repeated return demonstration. Certain procedures are still reserved for surgical or medical residents,
such as central line placement, chest tube insertion, or pulmonary
artery catheter placement.

As discharge approaches, patient follow-up is established with the
primary care physician and a dictated summary is forwarded regard-

ing the patient's hospital stay. Ongoing care management issues are investigated by a telephone assessment from the ACNP either with the patient or his or her physician. However, if the patient is not part of a primary care system, the ACNP facilitates a referral so that each patient she follows has access to ongoing medical care beyond the acute care episode.

Department / Unit Leadership

Because the ACNP is a master's prepared APN, she is a logical addition to the leadership group in her clinical setting. Clinical Nurse Specialists have historically been the source of clinical leadership for nurses in this institution and continue to provide staff support regarding expert nursing in areas of clinical specialization. Although CNSs are expected to spend a percentage of time providing bedside care, the nursing staff can be considered the client of the CNS because of his/her teaching and leadership responsibilities.

The leadership provided by the ACNP is also in large part educational, but with a different focus from that provided by the CNS. As is consistent with the preparation and practice of the ACNPs, they provide education about physical assessment and disease processes. Other leadership is accomplished by role modeling interdisciplinary cooperation and collaboration. The ACNPs are not involved in the aspects of leadership concerned with management of staff or employee supervision and evaluation. However, they are aware of the division issues and participate in problem solving as recognized nursing leaders. Because the patient, rather than the nursing staff, remains the principal client for the ACNPs, they must budget their time and energies accordingly. Investment of time in activities such as meetings has to be critically evaluated to provide enough time to adequately fulfill patient care responsibilities.

Acute care nurse practitioners are part of a hospitalwide leadership group of APNs. This group has a representative on the hospital council concerned with nursing practice issues, and is developing a statement regarding the scope of practice of APNs in the institution.

All departments where ACNPs are practicing have at least two branches of leadership, divided traditionally as "medicine" and "nursing." Due to this role's novel mixture of some traditional nursing duties with other responsibilities that were once considered to be in the province of medicine, the ACNP often receives leadership from both branches. The department financially supporting the ACNP usually maintains the dominant leadership and evaluatory role. It has been invaluable to have the backing of key members of nursing administration, regardless of which department financially supports the individual ACNPs. The relationship between the ACNP and head nurse is based on mutual respect and appreciation for the other's expertise in his or her professional domain. In addition to the nurse managers in each clinical area, having an advocate in central nursing administration who shares the vision of the role has been a valuable and necessary resource for advice and support.

Professional Development: Research, Publication, Presentations

In keeping with the term "advanced practice," the ACNP must support and promote ongoing research and publication of research outcomes for the expansion and enhancement of this role. This will add validity to the collaborative process with physicians and other health professionals involved at the bedside. Nursing science uses systematic inquiry to make change and redefine the way nurses think and practice. With the demand to change the way we think in health care, the ACNP role is a prime focus for research.

Expansion and development of this area of advanced practice will occur as new skills and expertise are scientifically tested and ethically evaluated. These new areas of research and development then encourage current practitioners to strive for the assurance of future change and integration of newer theories of advanced practice. This refinement cycle continues to take place in today's reformed health care system, increasing the visibility of the advanced practitioner. Increased visibility in the health care arena demands higher accountability. As innovative patient care systems emerge, advanced practice nursing is required to maintain accountability by employing the challenging process of inquiry.

Scientific evaluation of the ACNP role has begun as institutions like University Hospitals of Cleveland appraise the role in comparison to rotating house staff. The effectiveness of ACNP services needs to be measured by such outcomes as patient accessibility to the system, effectiveness of treatment, hospital resource use, and coordination of patient care across the continuum, including the transition out of the hospital. Controlled studies which isolate the effects of the ACNP role are difficult to carry out in the complex environment of tertiary-care hospitals, where patient care is provided by many different professionals. However, these evaluation efforts are essential to the continued development of the role.

Research also influences the ACNP's professional development by guiding advanced practitioners toward effective health maintenance, disease prevention, and rehabilitation of their patients. Once the inquiry process is tested and knowledge gained, it is up to credible experts to disseminate the outcomes to those it affects. This process not only benefits the patients and the institutions in which the ACNP practices but society as a whole. It is the ongoing process of research and exposure of data presented to appropriate audiences that begins to enhance the acceptance among physicians and consumers of the ACNPs as partners in care. Thus, participation in clinical research is an essential responsibility of all APNs, including ACNPs.

Participation in professional seminars and continuing education sessions, as well as publishing in professional journals, is another important aspect of professional development. This participation is essential in the arenas of both medicine and nursing. For example, ACNPs took part in a semiannual medical conference in Cleveland. The group presented the effective use of NPs in primary- and tertiary-care settings, an effort that exemplified the move toward greater physician acceptance and also professional development. The ACNP also teaches others preparing for advanced practice by conducting graduate level classes related to their area of clinical expertise.

As part of the ongoing professional development of this new level of practitioner, the ACNP group has realized the importance of addressing the lay public (in addition to professional audiences), educating these audiences regarding the qualification and abilities of ACNPs. The Cleveland ACNP group had the opportunity to inform the public about its role through the local media of television news and newspapers.

Teaching/Mentoring

All ACNPs have clinical faculty appointments at the university, associated with the hospital. They participate in precepting current ACNP graduate students in their clinical settings. Besides serving as a clinical instructor 2 to 3 days per week, the ACNP may teach one to two classes per semester. In addition, each ACNP is active in providing education for nurses and medical house staff with whom they work. Depending on the ACNP's area of expertise, he/she participates in hospital committees and projects pertinent to the level of advanced practice. However, committee involvement and teaching entails approximately 10–20% of the ACNP's overall responsibilities, in contrast to CNSs who may spend as much as 30–50% of their time in these endeavors.

For the nursing staff, the ACNP is able to provide access to current nursing and medical literature about the population specific to the patient division. Including information from the point of view that has traditionally been considered medicine serves to increase understanding about the rationale behind the medical plan. This, in turn, can help nurses teach patients about what is happening to them, improve nurses' clinical assessment skills, and contribute to the solidarity of the health care team.

For the interns and residents, the ACNP is an experienced resource concerning questions of management of problems unique to a particular patient population. The ACNP makes suggestions during daily rounds with the medical team, and the house staff observes how the ACNP manages patient problems. The ACNP can also help the house staff appreciate the value of interdisciplinary collaboration by acting as a liaison in formal and informal interdisciplinary meetings.

Each ACNP participates in teaching ACNP colleagues by giving educational presentations at the regularly scheduled monthly meetings. These presentations are on various topics that cross specializations, but are usually of special interest or reflect the clinical experience of the presenter. Subsequent discussions serve to problem solve, share experiences, and provide ongoing support within our peer group.

Variations and Implications of Differences

Integration in Various Care Delivery Models

Making the ACNP role fit well with the existing care models was challenging. Being considered a member of the medical team was awkward at first, but eventually ACNPs were accepted as valuable members of the team by physicians. Nurses also accepted the ACNPs, whom they found to be a new conduit for communication with the medical team.

In some areas, other new types of caregivers (PAs and case mangers) preceded the ACNP in the clinical setting. Acceptance of the ACNP may have been accelerated in these areas, as hospital staff already had experience with integrating various clinicians into the care delivery model. The other new types of caregivers performed a number of the same functions as ACNPs. It was important to explain and reinforce the differences between ACNPs and PAs and case managers. Recognition of the differences in educational background, breadth of preparation, and clinical experience is essential for the ACNP to function effectively on the team.

The presence of other new types of caregivers is a reality in the modern health care environment to which ACNPs must adjust. A number of factors lead to a potential for conflict in these working relationships. In interacting with PAs, sources of conflict include the somewhat competitive view with which both groups apparently have been socialized in their training. Large areas of overlap in the role responsibilities add to the potential for competition. Interestingly, each group seems to perceive the other as having more power, either institutionally or politically.

Differing education and backgrounds lead to understandable questions about which variety of clinician is more qualified than the other. ACNPs originate from a background that includes previous nursing experience. Educational preparation is a master of science in nursing, focusing on management of the acutely ill hospitalized patient. Physician assistants have many different types of backgrounds. Previous health care experience is often preferred but not required for PA educational programs. Types of educational programs offering PA content vary from associate degree preparation at a community college to university programs offering bachelor's or master's degrees.

Both ANCPs and PAs learn some degree of pathophysiology, pharmacology, physical assessment, differential diagnosis, and patient problem management. They also learn some skills and procedures. The most striking differences are based on the philosophical underpinnings of education for each type of clinician. The ACNP had nursing roots, while PAs arose from a perceived need within the traditional medical community and are educated to fill that need for a "physician extender". The PA role has undergone some evolution and is considered an independent profession now, though without a theoretical framework of its own (Jones & Cawley, 1994).

In the MICU, it was felt initially that the ACNP would be one of the "doctors." As time has passed though and the different disciplines have observed how the ACNPs are a mix of nursing and medical paradigms, they have come to be a group of their own rather than being grouped with either the "nurses" or the "doctors." This is beneficial in that both groups will often use the ACNP as a sounding board for ideas, plans, thoughts, or problems. In this manner the ACNP is able to actively influence the education of both nurses and doctors.

In the area of neuroscience, the ACNP has the opportunity to not only manage patients in the typical fashion for the acute care setting but to implement a new level of care coordination. The care coordinator role was developed for hospitalwide management of specific patient populations that are associated with standardized care paths according to admitting diagnosis. In addition to her or his individualized management of patients with various neurological diagnoses, the ACNP now acts as the care coordinator for patients carrying the diagnosis of ischemic stroke.

The ACNP redesigned the existing stroke care path to implement a case management model of care for the stroke patient. As often happens in large medical centers with multiple caregivers, specialists, and students, and with pressures to reduce length of stay, fragmentation of care and communication are major issues. This leads to redundancies as well as omissions in care due to unclear role responsibilities and patient goals. Use of care paths that had been developed was inconsistent without someone actually coordinating implementation. The ACNP had the opportunity to coordinate defined roles and outcomes already designated at expected time frames throughout the care path. Particularly with patients who have suffered strokes, needs are multidisciplinary and extend beyond the inpatient stay. The need for an extension of the stroke care path was identified and the care path modified to offer consistency throughout the rehabilitation period.

The ACNP often admits patients to the inpatient division once they have been seen and diagnosed in the emergency room by the neurology resident. The ACNP completes a standardized set of orders that was designed for the ischemic stroke patient. Patients are assigned a priority level that designates the severity of their stroke. The specific priority level activates the stroke care path. The ACNP can consult with the chief resident of the neurology service regarding unstable patient conditions. Ongoing management of anticoagulation and antihypertensive monitoring, as well as stroke risk management issues are handled by the ACNP. The ACNP, who works closely with social services, physical, occupational and speech therapy, prepares the patient for discharge. She also directs the monthly stroke support group offered to recovering stroke victims and their families.

The ACNP practice in adult internal medicine is independent of traditional models of patient care delivery in the tertiary-hospital setting. The Collaborative Clinical Service (CCS) health care delivery model operates on a 20-bed acute medical/surgical division. It is unique in that the care delivery team consists of two full-time ACNPs, a physician medical director, and the patients' private physicians, as well as division staff nurses. No fellows, resident physicians, house officers, or clinical nurse specialists participate in routine care delivery or patient management. The ACNP is geographically based on this division alone, providing care for the internal medicine patient population. Clinical practice involves direct patient management through a collaborative partnership with the patients' private physicians.

Patient management is as described previously in this text: history and physical exams, diagnostic reasoning, and therapeutic planning. The collaborative component to practice occurs with daily direct communication of patient condition and care design with his or her primary physician. Together the ACNP and physician make rounds at least once daily and communicate via phone as necessary. It is noteworthy that this type of care delivery requires increased communication and participation from the private physician beyond that traditionally required with house-officer models of care. Despite ongoing communication and collaboration, the primary physician retains the ultimate authority regarding patient management.

The ACNP has standard admission order forms from which to work in addition to specific protocols. Some protocols include heparin drip infusion, sliding-scale insulin regimens, and hypokalemia. Besides standard admission orders and protocols, interim orders in therapeutic planning result from direct ACNP-physician communication and collaborative decision-making efforts. Because of the lack of prescriptive authority in this state, all orders are written as verbal orders. They are carried out by the nursing staff immediately, and co-signed by an attending physician within 24 hours.

Overseeing the CCS as a medicine ward, the medical director serves as an immediate physician resource for both ACNPs and staff nurses. The relationship is highly supportive and designed in such a way that the ACNP may consult with him or her to review any patient case. The medical director's relationship with the staff nurses is one of resource as well as providing a backup for private physicians. For example, if the staff nurse is unable to contact the private physician on evenings or nights, the medical director may be called for assistance in solving patient issues. The problem may be addressed over the phone, and the patient's private physician then notified of the situation the following day.

In summary, the ACNP role responsibilities are similar but the individual ACNP has integrated the role to meet the needs of each clinical service, patient population, and clinical division. The ACNP role is adaptable and effective in each care delivery model, including working with PAs, working as part of a medical team, working as a care coordinator, and working as part of a team of ACNPs.

Patient Selection

Obviously the patients cared for by ACNPs are assigned to different clinical services. Even within one area, however, the question arises of which patients can be appropriately managed by the ACNP rather than by medical residents. The answer has come in part from the clinical characteristics of the patient group and in part from the characteristics of the clinical team.

Working with a very specific population of patients, such as on the oncology division, has resulted in a level of expertise in management of the problems faced by oncology patients. Continuity of care is also maintained for the patients who require frequent hospitalizations to the same division, allowing for chronic problems to be quickly addressed and incorporated into the plan of care. When a patient is admitted to the oncology division, he or she is assigned to an intern, a physician's assistant (PA), or the ACNP. This decision is made by some combination of the senior resident, the fellow, and the ACNP. Patients admitted for chemotherapy are almost always assigned to the ACNP or a PA. This allows patients to have the same caregiver each month as they return for cycles of treatment. The oncology division also cares for adults with sickle cell anemia, who have frequent admissions, and these patients also are usually assigned to the ACNP or a PA.

No patient is considered "too sick" to be cared for by the ACNP or a PA because of the strong collaborative design of the team. However, if a patient needs frequent orders throughout the night, arrives on the division after admitting hours for the ACNP, or requires a diagnostic work-up of particular interest, that patient is assigned to an intern. This practice reflects the fact that patient assignments are dictated not just by the acuity or stability of the patient, but also by organizational characteristics such as the ACNP and house officer staffing pattern.

Patient selection in the MICU is primarily based on clinical stability and diagnosis. Patients with critically unstable conditions, very unpredictable courses, those requiring frequent order changes during the night, or those of educational interest to the resident staff, will be assigned to the admitting resident of the day. Any other patient situation may be assigned to the ACNP. Examples of patients managed by the ACNP include diabetic ketoacidosis, gastrointestional bleeding, hepatic failure, asthma, chronic obstructive pulmonary disease exacerbation, myocardial infarction, and pneumonia. The entire MICU team makes rounds on all patients together and the ACNP is cognizant of all issues with all patients in the unit. As caseload permits, the ACNP will then assist the resident and nursing staff with management and technological issues of all the unit's patients. For example, the ACNP may spend time teaching and supporting a patient's family. Or perhaps he or she will review the hospital course of a particular patient for subtle factors that may have gone unrecognized and thus become contributors to the clinical decline. The ACNP will also assist with unit procedures. The ACNP inserts arterial lines, performs paracenteses and thoracenteses, draws blood, starts intravenous lines, trouble shoots technology, and assists the medical and nursing staff with interpreting data.

ACNPs in the MICU are unit based and often serve as a resource to patients for whom they have cared and their families, once they leave the unit. Calls are made to the ACNPs about follow-up plans, problems, or just for support. As much as possible ACNPs visit patients who have transferred out of the unit and evaluate the progress and implementation of discharge plans that were started in the MICU. The medical resident teams on the general divisions have become accustomed to working with the ACNPs and they occasionally seek assistance with issues.

The MICU ACNP generally works Monday through Friday during the daytime hours. As unit demands increase or decrease, hours may be extended into the evening or curtailed accordingly.

In the neuroscience setting, the ACNP admits patients with multiple sclerosis, seizures, Guillain-Barré, myasthenia gravis, and ischemic stroke. These patients are managed by the ACNP, with recommendations from the neurology chief resident, throughout the hospital stay. Patients who develop a hemorrhagic stroke and have been admitted by the ACNP are transferred to the neurosurgery service, with the ACNP then visiting them for continuity despite the service change.

Given the care coordinator aspect of the neurological ACNP role, the practitioner is committed to initiating a care path on all ischemic stroke patients in the hospital. This process is facilitated by the admitting department which faxes a list to the ACNP of all stroke patients admitted each day. The ACNP rounds on patients throughout the hospital, because stroke patients are often admitted by services other than neurology, such as internal medicine, family practice, and cardiology. When patients are on other services, ACNPs serve as a consultant, guiding patients through a path of care developed by those who specialize in stroke. Each ACNP manages an average caseload of 5–10 hospitalized patients at a time, admitting half of these under her or his service. Patients without private physicians, or those admitted to the staff neurology service, benefit most from the case management offered by the ACNP. ACNPs offer ongoing education, consultation, medication and anticoagulation management, often by telephone because it is difficult for them to cover the outpatient neurology clinic while managing inpatients. ACNPs follow the patient until he or she is attached to a consistent primary care physician. There are no specific ACNP-generated fees.

Differing from the population-based method of patient selection is the division-based method as it exists on the CCS. Here, patients are selected and admitted through project randomization or physician request. Patients originate from the emergency department, physician offices, admitting department, and outpatient clinics. All primary care medical patients ages 16 to 69 requiring hospitalization are eligible for admission. Those patients in need of specialty services, such as intensive care, neurology, or oncology, are excluded from randomization. The age-range determination was necessary because of a concurrent age-specific research project being conducted elsewhere in the hospital. The patients are randomly assigned to be admitted either to the CCS with ACNP care or to traditional hospital wards with house staff. This admission procedure provides a heterogeneous population for clinical comparison to traditional hospital-ward patient populations. Patient diagnoses vary widely, including conditions such as congestive heart failure, cellulitis/ osteomyelitis, asthma, pneumonia, obstructive lung disease, inflammatory bowel disease, diabetes mellitus, diabetic ketoacidosis (DKA), gastrointestinal bleeding, peptic ulcer disease, deep venous thrombosis, and pancreatitis.

Solo Practice vs. ACNP Team

Practice patterns of the ACNPs at University Hospitals of Cleveland vary somewhat according to the composition of the professional team. On divisions where there is one ACNP, assertion of the role is crucial to avoid homogenization with other types of caregivers who perform some of the same functions as the ACNP. It is common to be referred to as a PA by physicians, and in these cases it is important to call attention to the mistake, even if time only allows one to say "I'm an NP." In some cases, this statement will lead to questions about what the differences are between the roles. A brief description is probably most memorable in these situations, highlighting educational differences and nursing experience.

Common in most of the acute care settings is the presence of a CNS, head nurse manager, and possibly an assistant head nurse. This is true of the neuroscience area, where the ACNP functions interdependently as a nursing leader along with these individuals. However, the ACNP also functions quite differently from these individuals in terms of clinical management and patient care responsibilities, being the nursing presence among the physician's rounds and interdisciplinary meetings. This innovative level of advanced nursing practice has not only intrigued many of the physician members of the department of neurology, but has enhanced the partnership of care at the bedside for this population of patients.

The ACNPs on the CCS function as a team. They provide direct patient care that averages 12 hours per day Monday through Friday. As division demands and patient-care needs fluctuate, the ACNPs adjust the working hours accordingly. The framework schedule of the two ACNPs is four 10-hour workdays per week. This is managed by staggering shifts of 7:30 a.m. to 5:30 p.m. and 9:30 a.m. to 7:30 p.m. These shifts were established to enhance ACNP and physician availability for daily rounds together. Weekend days are without ACNP coverage at this time; therefore, patients' private physicians make rounds of their patients over these two days.

Admissions to the CCS service are structured according to the ACNP work schedule. Randomization of patients occurs Sunday night through Thursday evening including the hours of 5:00 p.m. to 11:00 p.m. Hospital statistics reveal that the evening and early morning hours contain the highest volume of admissions. Exclusion of these hours for patient randomization and admission forfeited a large number of patients for both research and ACNP practice. The departments of nursing and medicine arranged for patients to be randomized and admitted during these off hours by the "night float" physician—a resident whose function it is to admit patients from the hours of 11:00 p.m. to 7:00 a.m. The ACNP then assumes patient management the following morning. This arrangement represents one method to maintain an ACNP team census while also generating sufficient numbers of patients for the research project.

Another issue with ACNPs functioning as a team service is the need for evening- and night-shift patient coverage. On other services with ACNPs, patients are covered by on-call house staff. On the CCS, patient care issues on off-shifts are addressed in various ways at the discretion of the staff nurse. The staff nurse addresses patient needs with either a phone call to the private physician, instituting a protocol, or in an emergent situation, notifying the night chief resident (a senior resident on call in the hospital nightly). The protocols in use on the division were designed for both staff nurse and ACNP use. The protocols provide for timely therapeutic intervention for changes in patient condition.

Employing one ACNP to manage patient care for all ACNP "services" during night-time hours has been explored. The lack of prescriptive authority for NPs in the state of Ohio makes this option impractical and ineffective. Even if an ACNP were available to assess patient conditions, the physician would still need to be called for verbal orders. Off-shift patient management issues continue to be monitored and explored. In general, there are few patient issues/problems left unsolved by the time the ACNP leaves the division, and this issue has not been a significant problem.

With the varying methods of patient selection, patient welfare is still the paramount concern in organizing care delivery. The high acuity of today's hospitalized patient may necessitate interventions beyond the scope of ACNP practice. Our University Hospitals ACNP group believes a physician needs to be available for consultation regarding patient conditions. Incorporation of the ACNP into a medical team leads to the patient receiving the benefits of expertise from medicine and nursing in a collaborative partnership. Other options of house officer—ACNP teams may be worth exploring as well. ACNPs practicing in smaller community hospitals should have a physician available for consultative purposes either by phone or face-to-face communication.

COLLABORATION

In general the ACNP can encourage collaboration among members of the health care team by acting as a conduit of information between disciplines and encouraging individuals' participation in collaborating directly with other members of the team. The ACNP helps each discipline to realize the value and necessity of the others.

Nurses

Acceptance of the ACNP role among nurses seemed to occur after a period of testing and proving took place. Once nurses adjusted to the change of another caregiving role, a partnership focused on achieving patient goals began to evolve. A good example of this is the increased communication regarding patient care issues such as discharge planning. Patient discharge needs are assessed by the bedside nurse as well as the ACNP. Communication between ACNP, nurse, and patient enhances the speed and quality of discharge planning. This collaboration is illustrated by the case of a 52-year-old Black female who was admitted for her second stroke. Her past medical history included chronic atrial fibrillation and hypertension. Besides her antihypertensive medicines, this patient was also on long-term warfarin therapy. It was the admitting nurse who discovered that the patient stopped taking her anticoagulation medicine because of the cost. Considering her financial constraints and obvious need for continued anticoagulation therapy, the ACNP contacted the pharmaceutical company for its patient assistance program. This program allows indigent patients without Medicaid eligibility to receive needed medicine at no cost. With the help of the social worker and support from the attending physician, the patient was sent home and maintained on appropriate therapy.

In clinical areas where the ACNP is a member of the medical team, collaboration between nursing and medicine is enhanced. By being present at daily rounds the ACNP is familiar with every patient on the service. The nurses use the ACNP role as a communication liaison to underscore their patient care concerns to the physicians and to gain increased understanding about the medical plan of care. With current staffing patterns and level of patient acuity in the tertiary-care setting, it is difficult for the bedside nurse to maintain this level of ongoing collaboration with the medical team.

Residents / Fellows

In clinical areas with house staff, senior residents and fellows are valuable resources to the ACNP. Physician cosignature is required for orders written by ACNPs in the state of Ohio, and residents and fellows are usually willing to provide this. In cases where a difference of opinion exists on a question of patient management, discussion ensues and negotiation occurs.

In turn, the ACNP is a valuable resource for residents and fellows. Despite the presence of knowledgeable staff nurses, physicians sometimes exercise clinical decision making independent of other disciplines. With the advent of advanced practice nursing, physicians are challenged to collaborate with new partners in care. As the ACNP role has been incorporated into the medical team, physicians have come to appreciate the advanced practitioner who brings experience and knowlege to the collaborative process.

In a similar way, the roles of ACNPs and interns (first-year residents) are complementary. The ACNP, as a permanent member of the division, acts as a reference regarding patient care issues such as discharge planning, pain management, and individual patients' needs with which the ACNP may be familiar from past hospitalizations. The ACNP serves as a resource to the physicians in training as they learn the art of managing hospitalized patients.

Fellows who serve as consulting services throughout the hospital are a smaller group of physicians than the residents. They have come to know the different ACNPs on the various services and will often seek them out as a source of patient information. This mutually collaborative situation enhances relationships in the clinical setting. Since the ACNP is a member of the team who does not rotate off service and is knowledgeable about common patient issues, he or she may serve as a resource to consulting services and often serves as a conduit of information regarding the patient's plan of care and course. This is especially important to avoid fractures in continuity during the time the resident service changes.

Attending Physicians

Collaborative practice with attending physicians varies among the ACNPs in their clinical areas. The ACNP collaborates with both the patient's private attending physician and the attending physician of the hospital clinical service for the month. The ACNP directly manages the patient's care while the attending physician retains ultimate decision-making control regarding the therapeutic plan. Attending physicians vary in their efforts to micro-manage, often deferring judgment to the capabilities of the ACNP. The patient plan of care is developed through direct communication. The ACNP brings the art and science of nursing into the medical plan of care.

The ACNP also serves as a conduit to attending physicians who refer patients to the facility from outlying areas. The ACNP is careful to maintain regular communication with these physicians and update them on how their patient is progressing. Follow-up with these physicians is part of the discharge plan. This serves to remind all members of the health care team where the patients came from and where they may need to return.

Consultants and Referring Physicians

The Acute Care Nurse Practitioner practice incorporates the use of consultants from specialty services when developing patient plans of care. A formal consult is requested when the attending physician and ACNP seek assistance in further management of a patient's problems. The ACNP's involvement with consulting services promotes timely initiation of treatments and early evaluation of progress. When guidance from a specialty consult service is deemed necessary by the ACNP and the team, the designated resident on the consultation team will be contacted to present the patient's problem to him/her, as well as specific management questions regarding the problem. Relevant medical history and the specific questions about management are necessary to the consultation process. In addition to hastening the arrival at beneficial plan modifications for the patient, the interpersonal dynamics between consultation services and the medical team are optimized. When recommendations are made by the consultants, it is up to the ACNP and the other appropriate members of the team to incorporate the recommendations into the care plan. Often the members of the consultation team are able to provide valuable teaching to the ACNP and the rest of the team.

In some cases, residents on the consult services were hesitant to accept the request for assistance from an ACNP. They questioned the latter's ability to distinguish the need for specialty service and his/her authority to order the service. Over time, as more residents have become familiar with the knowledge and experience of the ACNPs, they have become more accepting.

Nurse Practitioners

Collaboration between NPs is evolving as the role evolves. Currently much informal consultation occurs between NPs in different specialty areas who possess needed knowledge and experiences. In addition, ACNPs collaborate with each other in efforts to teach the hospital community about the role. A formal consulting network is being established by the advanced practice group to facilitate this function.

The ACNP, as part of the medical team that remains on the division consistently, is in the position to maintain ongoing collaboration with the interdisciplinary team members, such as social workers, dieticians, home care coordinators, and physical therapists.

EVALUATION

Tracking: Documenting Volume and Quality of Service

With any new development and implemented change comes the need to evaluate the outcome of that change. So too, with the development of the ACNP role, one must establish a tool to measure change and the effects this role will have on patients and systems. It is only then that the transformation process can proceed. Visualizing accomplishments and productivity related to services rendered within this new level of care leaves the practitioner with a sense of gratification.

In the first year of practice as an ACNP, with its frustrations and distractions, many of the practitioners did not see the need for tracking data particular to their position. However, as time passed and performance evaluations were due, the need to capture quantity and quality of service became imperative. Some decided to track admissions, while others compiled data regarding types of procedures performed on a regular basis, success of those procedures, and patient outcomes.

More important as physicians begin to respond to the presence of NPs in settings where once only their counterparts practiced, documentation of patient satisfaction, quality improvement and fiscal benefit is necessary. An example of documentation activities can be found in the ACNP/care coordinator role in the stroke population. Here the ACNP maintains demographic information on each of the patients that are followed through the stroke care path. This provides a record for patient follow-up and telephone assessments that take place at 1 and 3 months postdischarge.

The ACNP completes a coded data sheet on each of the ischemic stroke patients being followed. This form tracks specific patient outcomes based on functional status before and after their care in the hospital, as well as outcomes of therapies, procedures ordered, and timeliness of discharge planning. Along with this inpatient evaluation, the ACNP tracks those patients who entered the system without a primary care physician. These data are important to note effects that ACNPs have on individuals without a consistent care system as well as referrals to community physician groups. The next level of tracking will include investigating discharge outcomes related to patients who were cared for under the guide of a critical pathway and care coordinator, and the effects of the care path on readmission.

CCS Project

A unique method of tracking patient outcomes, quantity, and quality of service is the prospective research project of the CCS, referred to earlier. The challenge of 20th century health care trends prompted this investigation of alternative methods of providing high-quality care with increased efficiency and cost savings. These trends include the current emphasis on ambulatory, primary care, projected decrease in federal reimbursement to hospitals for the cost of physician education, the continued escalation in costs of care at large medical centers, and the growing autonomy of professional nurses. In response, the care delivery system created in the CCS project "integrates traditional and advanced nursing functions [nurse practitioners] with physician functions ... As a result, the model is able to provide care to acutely ill patients but does not require resident physicians to function" (Collaborative Care, 1994).

The goal of the study is to evaluate the effect of collaborative care as an intervention in patient care delivery by measuring patient outcomes, hospital costs, and the organizational environment of care. The three elements characterizing this experimental unit are integrated patient assessment by doctors, nurses, and NPs aimed at reducing the duplication in traditional systems; nursing-initiated patient management, which expands the role of the nurses in assessment of acute patient problems using protocols; and patient-centered case management, designed for heterogeneous groups of medical patients, rather than for patients with a single diagnosis. These three elements are designed to increase efficiency and effectiveness of inpatient hospital care.

The CCS project was designed as a prospective controlled study of collaborative care over 3 years. As previously described, primary care medical patients are randomized to the collaborative care service or to a traditional hospital unit with house staff. Patient outcomes in the two groups will be evaluated based on several parameters. Traditional patient outcomes such as mortality and complication rate will be compared, as well as functional status, health status, symptom severity, and patient satisfaction. The project hypothesizes that the outcome status will be similar among the patients admitted to the collaborative care service and patients admitted to traditional medical wards.

The second aim of the project is to evaluate hospital resource use. Resource use is defined as hospital charges, length of stay, and estimates of actual hospital costs. The study hypothesizes that resource use will be lower in patients admitted to the collaborative care unit than in those patients admitted to traditional medical wards.

Lastly, the organizational environment of both units will be evaluated. The study hypothesizes that nurse-physician collaboration and the enhancement of the professional role of nursing on the collaborative care unit will promote nurses' job satisfaction and enhance the organizational environment of care (Landefeld, Rosenthal, & Brennan, 1992).

If the study hypotheses are confirmed this work will provide support for an alternative model of care that can be implemented and evaluated by other academic medical centers. In addition, this project is one avenue by which the APN can demonstrate efficiency of care and cost-effectiveness while maintaining availability of health care during demanding reform and hospital restructuring (Genet et al., 1995).

BARRIERS, BURDENS, BENEFITS

Throughout most clinical arenas there remains a consistent barrier to the ACNP's practice. Some members of the medical profession continue to perceive the ACNP as only a physician substitute attempting to assume more aspects of medical management. As ACNPs make efforts to gain acceptance from physician collegues, it becomes clear that most physicians are not familiar with the qualifications and capabilities of the NP. As on the CCS, the most effective method of education occurs when physicians actually admit patients to the ACNP service and experience the role first hand.

The uncertainty of some physicians regarding the newly developed ACNP role stems from multiplicity of titles that often describes various levels of advanced practice. ACNPs have often been addressed or introduced as nurse clinicians or PAs. Our discipline does not consistantly identify clinicians by their level of expertise, academic preparation, and practice setting. With all of the varying nomenclature, it is no wonder that physicians are reluctant to delegate shared levels of care. They are unsure of the nurse's clinical abilities because they do not recognize or understand the titles. This lack of identity impedes the collaborative process, especially in the acute care setting.

Along with this loosely defined role identity comes wide variation in expectations of members of the health care team. An example is the situation of a patient who has suffered a stroke and who requires a lumbar puncture. The ACNP is an expert in the care of these patients, has been thoroughly trained, and is experienced in the technique of lumbar punctures. The attending physician may believe that the ACNP is not qualified for this invasive procedure. Yet the fellow on the team may entertain the idea of having the ACNP perform the lumbar puncture, knowing this will save him from completing the procedure; the resident supports these efforts aware that the ACNP has already trained the medical students in the procedure. This inconsistency in expectations can lead to confusion, inefficiency in getting the work done, and frustration on the part of the ACNP.

Relationships with attending physicians can vary from collaborative partners in clinical practice to resistance toward the NP as part of the medical team. Certain physicians may turn a deaf ear to the ACNP's input on patient management issues. Resistance at the resident level comes with the resentment that the ACNPs do not take calls or cover their service after 8:00 p.m. in some settings or after 5:00 p.m. in others. It is also the resident or fellow who usually covers the ACNP's patients on the weekends. With this comes the laborious task of writing coverage progress notes on each of the ACNPs' patients and following plans that they have established. This poses a challenge to the medical paradigm and the subservient role that is traditionally imposed on nursing. In this case the resident may feel he/she is being asked to take a secondary role in patient care to the ACNP, and this can be perceived as a significant challenge to the physician's authority in patient management. It often seems that once a working relationship and rapport have been established between the ACNP and the physician group, one's identity has to be reestablished as soon as the new month begins and the residents rotate to another service.

Some common state-imposed burdens of the ACNP role include the areas of prescriptive privileges and direct reimbursement. Even from the mid-1960s on, as the NP role developed, there was controversy over the issues of state licensure. Although NPs saw themselves as diagnosing and treating patients, most state practice acts prohibited these actions, making major role components illegal. Eventually, by the 1970s, practice acts were rewritten to include these functions as well as language regarding prescription of therapeutic actions and medicines. Unfortunately, there is a wide disparity in the degree of prescriptive authority among states, and there are still four states without any legislative prescribing authority, including Ohio. Prescriptive authority is necessary especially if ACNPs are to participate in the health care market without a competitive disadvantage (Mahoney, 1988; Safriet, 1992).

Another major burden in offering effective advanced practice is the lack of the ability to be directly reimbursed for services rendered. While federal laws are slowly beginning to change, enabling some APNs to be directly reimbursed for their services, most are still paid by salary. Many NPs are not convinced that current salaries are sufficient compensation for the increased responsibility and accountablity in the health care system based on national averages of salaries of other advanced practice roles or even physician assistants. The American Nurses Association has advocated direct pay for nursing services since the 1940s; however, this was not significantly appreciated until now (Mittelstadt, 1993). Organized medicine has been opposed to direct reimbursement for APNs because it is perceived that this would allow them to practice independently, representing a direct threat to medicine's financial base.

Currently, in the retrospective cost-based system, NP services are billed under the physician charges or in agency fees. Unfortunately, insurers and legislators are unresponsive to reimbursement requests by yet another group of potential providers because they believe it will add to the inflationary health care dilemma. Here, NPs argue that separate reimbursement would allow the system to delineate contributions made by each provider and allow more accurate monitoring of actual costs. This is especially crucial in the costly hospital setting.

On the other hand, some of the benefits gained through the implementation of the ACNP role include the personal reward as well as the prestige and recognition associated with pioneering innovation in nursing practice. Despite some resistance initially, hospital administration offered support in the formalization of the ACNP position. Once fellow nurses had the opportunity to work with the new ACNPs and accepted their level of patient management, a new alliance developed at the bedside: nurses directing nurses in the clinical care of patients. Along with the responsibility of being a clinical expert on the division, the ACNP is seen as a leader among the staff.

Acute care nurse practitioner find there are many benefits to representing a specialty in their practice. Seasoned experience and advanced knowledge enhance their credibility among physicians and nurses. This allows the NPs to remain autonomous in their clinical decision making as well as complementing the collaborative process with all disciplines.

There is gratification in making advances in the legislative arena so that present and future practitioners can benefit from our actions and efforts. Working in partnership with clinicians who are changing the way they think about nurses' credentials and abilities at the bedside are exciting advances for our profession. Each practitioner carries the challenge of educating health care recipients of the value of this new role in the acute care setting.

A glance at the ACPNs' short history exemplifies their determination in changing the "status quo" of nursing care delivery. Representing the first ACNP graduating class, the honor of breaking new ground in health care is held in high regard within this group. The reformed hospital hierarchy of patient management in tertiary-level facilities is evolving rapidly. Advanced practice nursing remains an integral and vital component in the evolutionary process.

REFERENCES

Collaborative care: New vision for teaching hospitals. (1994, December). *Health care financing and organization news and progress.* Washington, DC: Alpha Center.

Genet, C. A., Brennan, P. F., Ibbotson-Wolff, S., Phelps, C., Rosenthal, G., Landefeld, C. S., & Daly, B. (1995). Nurse practitioners in a teaching hospital. *Nurse Practitioner, 20*(9), 47–54.

Jones, P., & Cawley, J. (1994). Physician assistants and health system reform: Clinical capabilities, practice activities, and potential roles. *Journal of the American Medical Association, 271*(16), 1266–1272.

Landefeld, C. S., Rosenthal, G., & Brennan, P. F. (1992). *A randomized trial of collaborative care: An alternative model for organizing health care delivery in teaching hospitals.* Robert Wood Johnson Grant proposal, unpublished.

Mahoney, D. (1988). An economic analysis of the nurse practitioner role. *Nurse Practitioner, 13*(3), 44–52.

Mittelstadt, P. (1993). Federal reimbursement of advanced practice nurses' services empowers the profession. *Nurse Practitioner, 18*(1), 43–49.

Safriet, B. S. (1992). Health care dollars and regulatory sense: The role of advance practice nursing. *Yale Journal on Regulation, 9*(417), 418–488.

Richmond, T. S., & Keane, A. (1992). The nurse practitioner in tertiary care. *Journal of Nursing Administration, 22*(11), 11–13.

INDEX

Springer Publishing Company

EXPERTISE IN NURSING PRACTICE
Caring, Clinical Judgment, and Ethics

Patricia Benner, RN, PhD, FAAN, **Christine A. Tanner,**
RN, PhD, FAAN, **Catherine A. Chesla,** RN, DNSc
Contributions by **Hubert L. Dreyfus,** PhD
Stuart E. Dreyfus, PhD and **Jane Rubin,** PhD

Based on the internationally renowned authors' major new research study, this book analyzes the nature of clinical knowledge and judgment.

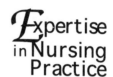

The authors interviewed and observed the practice of 130 hospital nurses, mainly in critical care, over a six year period. The authors collected hundreds of clinical narratives from which they refined and deepened their explanation of the stages of clinical skill acquisition and the components of expert practice. The text underscores the practical implications for nursing education and administration.

Partial Contents:

Introduction. Clinical Judgement. The Relationship of Theory and Practice in the Acquisition of Skill • Entering the Field: Advanced Beginner Practice • The Competent Stage: A Time of Analysis, Planning and Confrontation • Proficiency: A Transition to Expertise • Expert Practice

The Social Embeddedness of Knowledge. The Primacy of Caring, the Role of Expertise, Narrative and Community in Clinical and Ethical Expertise • The Nurse-Physician Relationship: Negotiating Clinical Knowledge Implications for Nursing Administration and Practice
1996 424pp 0-8261-8700-5 hardcover

536 Broadway, New York, NY 10012-3955 • (212) 431-4370 • Fax (212) 941-7842

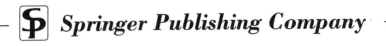

INCREASING PATIENT SATISFACTION
A Guide for Nurses

Roberta L. Messner, RNC, PhD, CPHQ
Susan J. Lewis, RN, PhD, CS

This manual guides nurses and others in the health care setting through the fundamentals of ensuring a satisfied "customer." It illustrates the many components of quality care, including how to provide clear and adequate information, create a hospitable environment, handle complaints efficiently, and design and utilize surveys of client satisfaction.

The authors draw from the principles of continuous quality improvement and other lessons learned from the business world, in addition to nursing's rich tradition of service. Written with warmth, sensitivity, and clarity, the book is an excellent resource for nursing students and practicing nurses. Health care institutions seeking good client relations will find this a suitable text for in-service training.

Contents:

What Do Patients Really Want? • The Changing American Healthcare Scene and Patient Satisfaction• Quality Isn't a Coincidence• Yes, Patients Do Have Rights • Patient Education: A Key to Increased Satisfaction • Creating a Hospitable and Healing Environment • How to Handle a Customer Complaint • Looking for the Lesson: Measuring/Evaluating Patient Satisfaction Findings • Be Kind to Yourself and Your Coworkers: A Plan for Enhanced Morale and Patient Satisfaction

1996   240pp   0-8261-9250-5   hardcover

536 Broadway, New York, NY 10012-3955 • (212) 431-4370 • Fax (212) 941-7842

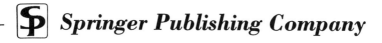 *Springer Publishing Company*

Nurse-Physician Collaboration
Care of Adults and the Elderly

Eugenia L. Siegler, MD, and
Fay W. Whitney, PhD, RN, FAAN, Editors

Foreword by **Joan Lynaugh** and **Barbara Bates**

Written by an RN-MD team, this book describes the current barriers to effective collaboration between nurses and physicians and suggests how to overcome them. Six successful examples of collaborative practice in a variety of settings are described. Specific guidelines for teaching collaborative skills to both physicians and nurses are outlined at length.

Today's health care trends are moving toward expanded use of nurse practitioners and other nurses with advanced training. In these circumstances, successful collaboration can mean better health care delivery for all.

Contents:

Springer Series on Advanced Nursing Practice
1994   264pp   0-8261-8500-2   hardcover

536 Broadway, New York, NY 10012-3955 • (212) 431-4370 • Fax (212) 941-7842

Springer Publishing Company

THE NURSE CONSULTANT'S HANDBOOK

Belinda Puetz, PhD, RN
Linda J. Shinn, MBA, RN, CAE

What is a consultant? What type of person makes a successful consultant? How does one launch and manage one's own business as a consultant? This manual answers these questions and provides comprehensive guidelines and practical information on becoming a nurse consultant. The authors, both experienced consultants, outline the consultation process in detail, describe the business and financial savvy required, and give tips on marketing and pricing one's services, making presentations, networking, and managing one's personal life in relation to one's career. The book addresses independent entrepreneurs as well as "intrapreneurs" who consult as an inside member of a larger organization.

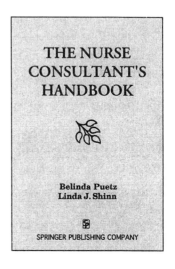

Contents:

- What is Consultation?
- The Consultation Process
- Preparation for Consultation: Planning a Career Path
- The Internal Nurse Consultant
- Starting a Consulting Business
- Marketing Consultation Services
- Networking
- Legal and Ethical Aspects of Consulting
- The Consultant as a Person

1996   280pp   0-8261-9520-2   Hard

536 Broadway, New York, NY 10012-3955 • (212) 431-4370 • Fax (212) 941-7842